The Importance of Being Sick

A Christian Reflection

by Leonard Bowman

A Consortium Book

Library of Congress Catalog Card No. 76-19774

ISBN 0-8434-0604-6

CONTENTS

To my Mother:
Margaret Hughes Bowman

FOREWORD

This book is simply a series of reflections on sickness viewed in the light of the Christian faith. It is frankly addressed to Christian believers, and uses the Christian Scriptures and the insights of Christian thinkers as tools for understanding a number of aspects of sickness and several problems connected with the care of the sick.

This is by no means intended to be a full-blown theology of sickness. It is not addressed to professional theologians. Nor is it in any sense a guide book for those who care for the sick. It is simply a series of reflections shared with anyone interested in pondering this painful but significant part of life. Hopefully it will be of some benefit to those who care for the sick, and especially to those who suffer sickness or similar painful human limitations.

These reflections are concerned with ideals, with what can happen in the life of a sick person animated by faith, or in the lives of those who serve the sick. A realistic awareness of the complexity and ambiguity of sickness and the care of the sick is to an extent presumed. The intent of this book is to provide a direction for thought, a framework of insights within which deeper meanings and richer possibilities might be discerned for the sick. Some of the problems and pains of sickness, however, point to a malaise within our society, an apparent inability to face sickness and death. And so while we reflect on the meaning and possibilities of sickness, we will find ourselves raising questions about the good health of our culture, too.

I would like to express my appreciation to all who have helped me, directly or indirectly, in the writing of the book.

The faculty and students of Nursing at Marycrest College, Davenport, Iowa, provided me with many insights, often unknowingly. Sr. Michelle Cale, O.S.F., R.N., of Mt. Marty College, Yankton, South Dakota, helped in clarifying my ideas and offered constructive advice on the manuscript. Sr. Mary Helen Rappenecker, C.H.M., of Marycrest College, aided me in preparing the manuscript for publication. Thanks to the editors of the *Saint Anthony Messenger* for permitting me to include parts of my articles, "Theology of Death" and "Theology of Sickness." And I am especially grateful to my wife Anne for her continuing help and encouragement.

Davenport, Iowa
December 15, 1975

Part I

The Sick and Health

Reflections on sickness begin by pondering what sickness means, first in our everyday commonsense world, then in the Christian Scripture. The first leads to the conclusion that sickness needs to be understood and accepted as part of life. The Scriptures reveal a profound significance in the sickness that is accepted in a spirit of faith and hope.

Chapter 1
What is Healthy?

One of the more annoying jokes that our language plays on us is to let us think that we know for sure what certain common words mean. "Sick" and "healthy" are words like that. Everyone knows what it means to be sick, and what it means to be healthy is even more obvious. But how easy is it to say just what these words mean?

The nastiness of this joke becomes apparent whan a person starts to *question* the words, and to *wonder* about what they mean. It is nasty first because of the kind of reaction we get when we ask something like "what does it mean to be sick?" People look at us if we're sick or something. If they do eventually take you seriously, they'll cough up a lame answer like "Sick is—you know—like feeling lousy," or "Sick? When something's bothering you." That gets nowhere, because we know we can be perfectly healthy—whatever that means— and still feel lousy because things still bother us.

But the nastiest thing about this joke is that because of it we seldom stop to question and wonder at all the obvious things that make up much of the real substance of life. And so we tend to skate merrily along like water bugs on the thin, deceptive surface of living, and never think to let ourselves be immersed in its depth. Until something disturbs that surface, that is: then there's a chance of drowning in what seemed so obvious.

But if a person is willing to risk belaboring the obvious or admitting ignorance about what everyone knows, he sets out

3

on a voyage of discovery and begins to probe the deep currents of significance that stir beneath most obvious things, beneath health and especially beneath and within sickness.

What does "sick" mean? What does "healthy" mean? A dictionary should have something to say about that. But dictionary definitions of obvious things are quite a joke: they lead you in circles:

Sick (sik) adj. 1. Suffering from disease or illness. Check "disease":

disease (di·zēz) n. 1. Any departure from health. Check "health":

health (helth) n. 1. Freedom from defect, pain, or disease. The dictionary tells us what we knew already: sickness and health are defined in terms of each other. Then either the meanings of "sickness" and "health" are obvious, or maybe sickness and health are incomprehensible.

The dictionary has, however, given authority to the obvious, commonsense knowledge that sickness and health are opposites. Sick means not healthy, and healthy means not sick. Sickness and health are mutually exclusive.

Health is obviously good, a desirable condition. And so sickness is bad, something to be avoided or prevented. Or, if by some bit of bad luck it is too late for that, sickness is something to be cured, gotten rid of. To be sick means to *be* in an undesirable, bad condition, to be for a time what is to be avoided or prevented or cured.

Get Well Soon

What happens when this commonsense understanding of sickness is seen in the larger context of a person's life as a whole, or in the context of the business of living in American society?

One of the things that happens is the get-well card.

The get-well card provides an opportunity to penetrate beneath the obvious, for it is a gesture. Like most gestures, it embodies and expresses—sometimes eloquently—an unspoken and even unconscious attitude. And unspoken attitudes often have deep roots.

An important dimension of this gesture is that it is usually made by the healthy toward the sick. It expresses then, among other things, what sickness means to the healthy person engaged in the business of living in American society.

What is the unspoken thing that the get-well card says?

For the sake of scientific objectivity, we need to examine a random sample of get-well cards. A selection from the greeting-card rack of a Schlegel-Rexall drug store in the middle of Davenport, Iowa, should be random enough for our purposes.

The first specimen has blue forget-me-nots, watercolor style, on a pale yellow background. Inside the verse says,

> Hope it won't be long at all
> Until the day's at hand
> When you're enjoying perfect health
> And really feeling grand.

On the back it says "35 cents."

The comic cards for the most part envision a healthy sex life between the (male) patient and the nurse. An exception pictures an obviously miserable hospital patient abed under a mountain of covers and crowned with a hot-water bottle. Next to the bed is a fully-equipped bedside stand—complete with bedpan. "Bet you'll be glad to be out of there . . ." it threatens. Inside, ". . . and on your *own* again," with a picture of a toilet. That one costs 50 cents.

An instructional one lectures on "Three reasons for getting well soon" beneath a cover of pastel sweet peas. The climactic third reason declaims,

> You ought to get well
> So you can find
> Through carefree days ahead
> The happiness that you deserve.

There is something to hope for—but don't hold your breath.

A white colonial church pictured against a misty pink and

purple sky offers spiritual comfort. "Praying for your recovery," announces the cover. Inside it prays,

> Since God hears every prayer that's said
> And knows our problems, too
> Then brighter days and better health
> Are just ahead for you.

So we discover that religion can provide an interesting variation on the fortune cookie. This one is also 50 cents.

These are the kinds of things get-well cards say in addition to "get well soon." But what is unspoken?

Imagine these cards on the bedside table of an accident victim who faces a hospital stay of two months or more, perhaps much of it in traction. What do they say to him, just beneath the surface?

"Hope it won't be long at all . . . ," but everyone knows it will be long, and it may be questionable if the sick person will *ever* enjoy "perfect health" again.

"Bet you'll be glad to be out of there. . . ." It would probably be a sure bet. That suggests, though, that the odds are very high against anyone ever having reason to be glad to be *in* there. And so the card tells the sick person to shift his thoughts to that indefinite future day of absolute liberation, the day he can return to his very own toilet.

Another card from our random sample offers that advice in so many words. It pictures two happy watercolor children romping with bunches of pastel balloons through billowy grass and blurry bright flowers. It suggests,

> Hope the hours will hurry by
> While you must stay in bed
> And that your thoughts will center on
> Much brighter days ahead.

Yes, dream yourself away from where you are and into a pastel and flowered future. For a person who faces only a few hours of sickness, such advice might be appropriate. But for our accident victim, it seems grotesque. It would do less to console than to make him impatient with his lot.

The unspoken message of the other two cards cuts deeper. ". . . Get well, so you can find through carefree days ahead the happiness that you deserve." The first suggestion beneath the surface here is that the patient obviously cannot be happy being sick. That is logical, of course, because according to the commonsense notion sickness is undesirable, so that only healthy people can be happy. The second suggestion is that happiness is necessarily connected with being carefree— without pain, disappointment or struggle. The third suggestion is that this carefree happiness is something you *deserve*. Cares, struggle and sickness are then undeserved, unjust and unfair. Our accident victim should therefore feel put upon, resentful, and even angry. The pastel sweet peas inadvertently counsel rage and rebellion!

The sweetest counsel of all comes from the little white church. God is good and kind and loves us, and therefore "brighter days and better health are just ahead for you." Our accident victim knows only too well that "just ahead" underestimates the time by quite a bit. He knows too that worse days are more likely. Then the logic of this gentle prayer suggests that God must not be good and kind, or if he is, he doesn't care about us. Or maybe he just can't *do* anything about it! The suggestion is that God is malevolent, unconcerned or ineffectual—and so the consoling message turns bitter, echoing subtly in its implied despair the kind counsel of the sweet peas.

But the most pervasive and perhaps the cruelest unspoken attitude is embodied in the most obvious message spoken by every such card: "Get well soon." Our accident victim is not about to get well soon, and he knows it. Then what are all these cheery gestures conveying to him, unspoken, from his healthy friends? "Get well soon," and get back into the business of life. "Get well soon," because there's nothing to do in your present situation, no use or value at all in how you are living now. "Get well soon," because there is no chance of happiness for you until you do. For while you are *there*, in your sickness, there is nothing we can offer you, say to you, or share with you. While you are sick and we are healthy, you just don't fit anywhere in our lives at all. You are in an undesirable condition, to be avoided or ignored unless you are cured quickly. After all, sickness and health are mutually exclusive, even according to the dictionary. If you are sick, you're out of it.

The get-well card seen as a gesture, then, conveys a very discouraging message to the sick. It is of course an unspoken message, and one would assume that the attitude it expresses is quite unconscious. After all, people just don't feel that way about those they send get-well cards to.

Of Course, That's Just Something People Say

Perhaps then we are reading the gestures of the get-well card too seriously. It is simply a convention, a convenient way of expressing concern. People don't mean get-well cards literally—cards say the sort of things cards are supposed to say, taken-for-granted things.

This is a consoling thought, especially if our wonderings so far have led any hapless get-well-card receiver to suspect the intentions of the people who sent those cheery greetings. And it is undoubtedly true that such unkind thoughts are the farthest things from the senders' minds.

But the unspoken, unconscious attitude is there all the same, implicit in the gesture. The attitude is built into the conventional taken-for-granted things that people say to a sick person, and that a sick person accepts at face value. It is *there*—but no one seems to notice.

This is not a consoling thought. It is *alarming*.

Why is "get well soon" the thing people say? Considering its implications at least for a chronic or long-term patient, it doesn't make the best sense. But it has a certain cogency, a certain fitness—enough at least so it can be taken for granted. And it can be taken for granted because it does fit into all the other things everyone takes for granted—the whole set of assumptions, habits, and expectations that are so built into our culture that they have become second nature. What is taken for granted is something so close or so pervasive that no one gives it a thought.

That is what is so alarming.

What is the place given to sickness within the assumptions, habits, and expectations that make up our contemporary American culture?

In the media, quite a lot of attention is given to *cures*. There are pills advertised for every pain. News reports and television series proclaim the heroic strides of white-coated physicians and scientists in the valiant march to discover or develop cures for every known illness.

One obvious place that is given to sickness is the hospital. But the hospital too is pictured as a place for sickness to be cured. Sirens scream and red lights flash and there is a state of emergency, but if you get to the hospital everything will be all right. You will "get well soon."

But what place is made in the business of living in American society for *being sick*? Does the sick person have a place, or is he "out of it"—at least until he gets well?

Hospitals can also serve as attractively-landscaped repositories where people who are *being sick* can be placed out of the way, where they will be "all right": so the generality of healthy persons need not concern themselves about the sick and can be about the business of living unencumbered.

Another get-well card from our random sample reinforces this idea of the place given to being sick:

> It seems a shame that anyone
> But especially *you*
> Should have to spend a single day
> Feeling the way you do.

Sickness is a shame, and being sick is out of place. There is no room for sickness in our busy consciousness. If you must be sick, hide it. Pretend you're perfectly healthy. Or else hide yourself away, separate yourself from the healthy so that you won't disturb our way of living. Oh, but do get well soon.

In Pursuit of Paradise

Being sick, then, doesn't really seem to have a place among the assumptions, habits, and expectations that make our contemporary American culture. It doesn't really fit into the pattern formed by the things we take for granted.

Perhaps a critical look at that pattern would help to make it clear why.

Advertisements are a good indicator of commonly held assumptions and expectations, for ads deliberately capitalize on the unspoken, probably unconscious convictions and desires that move people to act.

Here is a picture of an exquisitely healthy-looking young couple, obviously in love, skipping with pastel balloons through billowy grass and flowers. Balanced on their ecstatically parted lips are cigarettes. Unbounded joy and happiness is sold in packs of twenty, if you allow the mystical vision of the advertiser to set your expectations. Of course, people are more sensible than that.

A dress, to judge from its setting and from the expression of the model who displays it, offers unimpeachable prestige in high society. A particular brand of whiskey offers the experience of unmitigated success. By driving a particular car, one is to discover the height of human fulfillment. A particular house on a secluded lane offers a private Eden. And if you don't find it there, your travel agent beckons you to "pleasure yourself in Paradise"—in a wide selection of paradises, as a matter of fact.

Of course, people are too sensible to fall for all that. That's why they smoke the cigarettes, buy the dresses, select the whiskey, make incredible payments on the car, fly to the overpriced and overcrowded shangri-la, and move to the suburbs.

It is a strange but pervasive game, this chasing of rainbows, this pursuit of paradise. Everything offers the state of "having arrived," but never quite meets the game's pattern of expectations. One never arrives. The reality never meets the expectations.

It would seem logical to alter the expectations.

But what actually appears to be happening in the game is that the expectations dictate certain alterations in the reality—or at least in the awareness of reality.

The game demands that the one who plays it develop the capacity to act *as if* they have arrived in an earthly paradise. This capacity has two aspects. First is a studied effort to create the image by trying to look like that ecstatic young couple in the cigarette ad, while telling yourself you really feel that way. (Imitating the whiskey ad is easier, of course, because the props help to foster the illusion.) The second aspect is an extremely thorough campaign to ignore or hide anything that casts a shadow on the image. If the player masters this capacity, he can win the game by absolutely convincing himself that he is indeed a perfect man living in an earthly paradise where everything is beautiful and nothing is ugly. If something is ugly, ignore it. Move to the suburbs. If even there something ugly props up, like a small boy chasing a baseball through your petunia patch, holler to the authorities, whose task it is to set things right and make the American Dream invulnerable. And if there is something ugly that can't be set right, at least we can devise some effective method of hiding it.

Sickness? Not here, no—we can't have that. Sickness would mess up the image. If you *insist* on being sick, of course, we'll simply have to hide *you*. At least until you get well.

> . . . a shame that anyone
> Should have to spend a single day
> Feeling the way you do.

Firm Ground

Playing this game, the pursuit of paradise, demands such an effort not to see things that it would seem discouraging to most people, and few indeed would be expected to keep it up for long.

It is alarming then to see that this game, this "American Dream" is in many ways so close and so pervasive that it is second-nature to us, and no one gives it a thought. It is the unspoken, unconscious attitude that governs our choice of cigarettes, whiskey and places of residence, and perhaps that lies at the root of our penchant for sending get-well cards.

Our questioning and wondering about those obvious things, sickness and health, has led us to probe beneath the commonsense notions, and to discover the deep assumptions and attitudes in which those notions are rooted. What we have discovered is a strangely illusory game, a dream, that floats beneath the surface of our culture. And we are disturbed to find ourselves caught up in this game even in spite of ourselves.

We are like the person having a nightmare who comes out of the dream just enough to know it is a dream, but for all his willing and his effort cannot wake up. The dream holds him, captivates him, and becomes the more terrifying the more it seems inescapable. And when he wakes, startled, he feels about him, looks hard into the darkness about him to find reassuring reminders of reality, so as to convince himself that the nightmare was indeed a dream.

But when the dream is so widely shared and pervasive, reinforced by all the props and sets we have built to maintain the illusion, where can we find genuine reminders of reality?

Perhaps rescue can be found by looking hard into those things that the game makes such an effort not to see. Sickness, for example.

We need to ask once again the deceptively simply question, "What does it mean to be sick?" "What does it mean to be healthy?" Then we need to probe the deep currents of significance that stir beneath sickness seen as a reminder of reality, to see what image of life, what set of attitudes emerges when a person does give a place to sickness, and make room for it in his consciousness.

The commonsense understanding of sickness and health as

opposed, as mutually exclusive, has been tested. We found that it had shallow roots.

Another meaning that the dictionary gives to the word "healthy" may provide a better path to understanding. It is, simply, "sound." That in turn means "solid; whole and in good condition." *Whole.* To be healthy is to be whole, to be in one piece, to have integrity.

What happens when this understanding of health is seen in the larger context of the business of living in American society?

For someone to have a healthy life would then call for him to make of all the bits and pieces of that business an integrated whole. It would call for him to live in a way that takes every aspect of life into account. It calls for an image of life, a set of attitudes that gives place to every aspect of life, and makes of life a unified sense, a harmonious whole.

For someone to have a healthy life would then call for him to take sickness into account, and give a place to it that allows sickness to contribute its significance to the meaning of his life.

If this understanding of health is true, then the common-sense notion of health as *excluding* sickness appears to be positively *unhealthy.* Real health, wholeness and integrity, has to include and embrace sickness within its harmonious integration of the business of living.

And if this understanding of a healthy life is true, then the whole image of life and set of attitudes connected with the dreamy pursuit of paradise appears to be radically sick. To live is not to be a pair of ecstatic, cigarette-balancing manne-quins romping through billowy grass and pastel flowers. Sickness and other reassuring reminders of reality suggest that living includes suffering pain, confronting the ugly and dealing with it honestly, and going through the bumps, frustrations and struggles that are part of the process of growth, change, and deepening. Real living is not to "have arrived;" it is to be *on the way.*

To Your Health

An understanding of health as wholeness can make quite a difference in our attitudes toward a person who is occupied with *being sick*. Perhaps it can provide a corrective to some of the well-intentioned but misguided counsel offered by our random sample of get-well cards.

Surely no one would wish a long hospital stay on someone, and so it would be in place to "bet you'll be glad to be out of there." But if sickness is an integral part of life's process of growth, change and deepening, then perhaps the sick person can find a reason to be happy in this present challenge to live more deeply. And perhaps his sickness will offer him an opportunity to discover or develop a sense of liberation that is a bit more spiritual than the ability to return to his own toilet.

If a reason for wanting to get well is "so you can find, through carefree days ahead, the happiness that you deserve," perhaps a healthy attitude toward sickness could help a sick person to find a more realistic happiness. If sickness and pain are expected, taken into account as an integral part of living, then there is no cause for impatience or resentment. If indeed sickness is a force that brings growth and deepening, then perhaps the days ahead—while not carefree—will lead him to a new depth of happiness.

And if real health includes and embraces sickness, then the sick person is very much engaged in the business of life. He has an extremely significant mission to do, and there is profound value in what he is doing. And while he is there in his sickness, he has a vital aspect of life to offer to others and share with them. Indeed the thoughts of the sick person and of those who love him should not "center on much brighter days ahead," for playing that game poisons a person's ability to develop a healthy awareness of the meaning of what he is doing in the present, *while* he is sick.

Perhaps then "Get well soon" and the gesture it implies could well be replaced by a wish that the sick person may *be* healthy, even in his sickness.

An understanding of health as wholeness, then, should result in attitudes of appreciation, respect, and sharing between the sick and the physically healthy. What the sick person does has value, for it is an integral part of life. Perhaps it is such an understanding of the meaning of sickness within an integral Christian life that lies behind a very odd thing said by St. Francis of Assisi. His little company of friars had all been disgustingly healthy for a year, and Francis was heard *complaining* that they had not had any "blessing" that year: no *sick* friars!

But health understood as wholeness is not something that just happens. It implies a whole style of life, just as the commonsense notion of sickness and health as opposites implies the dreamy game of pursuing paradise. Where do we find the focus of that style of life, the deep center around which the many aspects of life gather to form an integral whole?

This question probes the currents of significance that stir beneath the surface of sickness, and calls us to discover the depth of life which sickness can reveal.

Chapter 2

Sickness Means Something

The obvious place for Christians to look as they seek the significance of sickness is in their Christian faith, especially in its expression in the Scriptures. This is an obvious place to look for enlightenment, but as with most obvious things, the surface of the Christian faith is deceptive, and the Scriptures can play jokes just as language can, tricking us into thinking we understand for sure what certain words, stories, practices, or teachings mean.

Once again, a person has to be willing to risk belaboring the obvious or admitting that the Christian faith he claims to live is something he does not fully understand. Then he can set out on a voyage of discovery and probe beneath the surface to the deep currents of significance that stir in the words, stories, practices, and teachings of his faith. He has to try to discern the pattern formed by apparently disconnected comments on a theme such as sickness, and discover—by allowing the Scriptures to speak to *him*—the unspoken meaning that is there just beneath the surface, implicit in the encounter between a believer and the expressions of his faith.

One trick that the Bible can play on us is to tempt us to seize on a particular passage that teases us with the promise of meaning and to cling to it without seeing it in the context of the whole of the Bible and the whole of the Christian life. Taken out of context, the words of Scripture can be deceptive—indeed there is much sense in the old saying that even the devil can quote Scripture to his own purposes.

At the very least, there are many different ways in which people understand such basic Christian ideas as sin, repentance, grace, and salvation, and such basic Christian realities as Christ, the Cross, the Church, and sacraments. As a result, in the attempt to talk about these things, we have to make a special effort to avoid confusion. So as we look at what the Christian Scriptures have to say about sickness, we will be concerned about understanding those words, stories, practices, and teachings in terms of the whole of the Christian life.

The Christian faith in a nutshell

In order to understand clearly the context for Christian ideas about sickness, perhaps we had better take the time for an overall view of the Christian faith. Admittedly, we can do only a "once-over lightly" reflection, limiting our perspective to the way a person might live his Christianity.

What then does it mean for a person to be a Christian?

Deep within every person—in fact at the core of every person—is a yearning for meaning, for wholeness, for enduring value. That yearning leads a person on a lifelong quest, as he seeks his meaning consciously or unconsciously in heaven knows how many different ways. Some try to find themselves in a career, some in fame, some in wealth, some—luckier than the rest—in a relationship of real love for another person. But none of these ways give a meaning that is beyond a doubt, a wholeness that is truly complete, or a value that really endures. And so left to himself, a person discovers that he cannot fulfill his yearning, and his quest is hopeless . Every merely human effort to find meaning is ultimately frustrated by the universal law that all living creatures suffer and die, and all monuments erode and decay.

Man left to himself is hopeless, and the yearning for meaning at his core is a useless passion, leading only to despair.

Maybe we could say that the state of *sin* is the condition of a person left to himself, hopeless and alone. He faces the inevitable and absolute reign of death and decay with whatever Stoic calm, cavalier nonchalance, or just plain rebellion he can muster. Or perhaps we can say that the state of sin is reflected in the effort of people to create the illusion of a paradise on earth, forgetting or ignoring both the rule of death and the call of God.

And yet there is a realm where death is not absolute. There is one who is not subject to death and decay, but who gives life. There is one who is meaning, who is wholeness, who is the enduring ground for all value. There is one who is in himself the goal of a person's quest for meaning. To speak of him men use the word "God."

But how can a person reach God?

Left to himself, a person cannot reach God. If he could, then mankind would have in itself the power to reach beyond death. And we know that this is not the case. God is transcendent: he is beyond the reach of human powers, as well as beyond the reign of death.

But God can reach to humankind and form a relationship—much like love—with persons and with peoples. He doesn't have to. If he does form a relationship with humankind, he does so freely, gratuitously. And of course such a relationship with God would in itself give a person a meaning beyond limit, a wholeness that is absolutely complete, and a value enduring as transcendence. Because it would be absolutely gratuitous, such a relationship with God would be called "grace."

The Old Testament testifies that God did indeed reach to humankind, and formed a relationship or covenant with a people he freely chose to be his own. His steadfast love preserved that relationship in spite of failures on the part of man. So in that chosen people God planted and fostered the seed of his own realm where death is overcome.

Jesus Christ bears witness that God's reaching out to humankind is absolute, universal, and irrevocable. In Jesus Christ the realm of God—the Kingdom of Heaven—is definitively established. In him the relationship between God and humankind is perfectly and completely realized—so perfectly in fact that God and man are made one in the unity of a single person, Jesus. Jesus Christ *is* God's reaching out to men, and he *is* at the same time man's response to God. He *is* God's free gift of loving union with men, and so we might say that he *is* the reality of grace.

Jesus definitively established the realm of God and so founded once and for all the stable relationship between God and men by his Crucifixion and Resurrection. In this Paschal or Easter mystery he overthrew the realm of death, and passed over with all mankind to the realm of God. So with him all humanity was given a way to freedom from that realm where a person is left to himself in despair, a way into the realm of God, the reality of grace, where a person can discover the free gift of God's love.

Maybe we could say then that the state of grace is a vital relationship between man and God, a relationship that Jesus Christ has established and that he embodies. And the state of sin is estrangement from God, the ignoring or refusing his free gift of love.

When Christ began his public life, his message was "repent and believe the good news." The good news was that God's kingdom was being definitively established, that God was reaching to all mankind with an absolute and irrevocable love. To repent meant simply to turn from a state of sin to the state of grace: to let go of the desperate attempt of man to find meaning on his own, and to accept the relationship with God that is freely offered in Christ.

How does a person act out that repentance and live out that relationship with God? How is a person one with Christ?

Two images from the New Testament shed light on the relationship between Christ and the person who believes in him, who accepts the relationship with God that is offered in him. The Gospel of John speaks of a vine, and the epistles of Paul speak of a body.

Believers are to Christ as branches to a vine. Note, not as branches to the trunk of a vine, but to the vine itself. Where would the vine be without the branches? It wouldn't exactly

be a vine! Christ and those who believe in him form a single
organic unity: as a community, believers are one reality with
Christ. As Paul describes it, their unity is the organic wholeness of a body, each member distinct and making a unique
contribution, yet nothing apart from the whole. The *whole*
Christ is the organic unity of Christ and believers.

That is the fundamental reality we call "Church." It is the
organic unity, the community of believers in Christ. A person
lives out his relationship with God and his unity with Christ
through participating in the Church.

But participation in the fundamental reality of the Church
is not quite the same thing as being a collection-paying
member of a particular congregation or parish. That is on the
surface, and there is plenty of evidence available to indicate
that it can be an empty show. What gives authenticity and
meaning to being a member of a parish or congregation is the
participation in the fundamental reality of the Church which
such membership is supposed to express and symbolize. It is
this organic oneness with Christ which is acted out and
embodied by those who share the sacramental community
meal of the Eucharist. It is this participation in Christ's
triumph over the reign of death by his Cross and Resurrection
which is acted out and made real by those who share in the
Easter sacrifice of the Eucharist.

A person acts out his repentance, and so abandons an
isolated and estranged state of being and accepts the relationship with God that is offered in Christ, by baptism. Baptism is
not quite simply an initiation ceremony, trickling a few drops
of water over a person's head. That is on the surface, and
sometimes that is as deep as it may reach in a person. What is
acted out and made real in baptism is a person allowing
himself to be plunged into the reality of Christ (*baptizare*
means "to plunge"), to be immersed in Christ and so made
one with him. And it is a person plunging down into the realm
of death as Christ did in dying, and emerging victorious as
Christ did in rising, so entering the reign of Christ and
participating in the Kingdom of God.

Christ sent his followers into the world, which was yet unrepentant, as his Father had sent him—to witness that God's reaching to humankind is absolute, universal, and irrevocable, and to incorporate the world as a whole into the reality of Christ (the vine, the body). The hope of believers is for the universal completion of the kingdom of God which has been established in Christ, as Paul the Apostle said, for "all things to be reconciled through him and for him, everything in heaven and everything on earth" (Col. 2:20). In its fundamental reality, then, the Church is on its way, embodying Christ and making his presence manifest through human history, while struggling and hoping for the completion of Christ's kingdom.

In a nutshell, then, being a Christian means participating by faith in the reality of Christ through his Church, and consequently living in a way that reflects Christ and bears witness to his good news. To the extent that a person does so share in Christ, then in every detail of his life Christ is embodied and made real. Speaking as such a member of Christ, Paul described his life this way: "I live now not with my own life but with the life of Christ who lives in me" (Gal. 2:20). And what he describes is not some saintly mysticism of an elite, but the fundamental everyday reality that every Christian lives, however much or little he is aware of it. To be a Christian is to participate in Christ.

Within Christian life understood in this way, what is the place of sickness?

What the Bible says about sickness

If we take a close look at what the Bible has to say about sickness, we discover quite a variety of ideas, and not all of them would fit well into the Christian life as we have described it. But what the Bible describes is a history: the history of God's reaching out to humankind. In that history there has been quite a lot of development, especially in men's understanding of what it means to be God's people.

One aspect of that development concerns how people came

to cope with sickness. The different ideas about sickness show a real deepening of men's understanding of their own suffering, and a gradual awakening to the meaning of their suffering in their relationship with God. These ideas show a real growth through history.

/ ,   In the earliest stage of that development, sickness was looked upon as God's punishment for sin, and God's vengeance upon evildoers. The covenant relationship between God and his people was expressed in the Law of the Old Testament. If a man were faithful to that Law, then he could expect health and prosperity as a reward. If he were unfaithful, then God would punish him with sickness and misfortune. The first psalm expressed how a faithful Israelite expected to be treated by his God:

> Happy the man
> who never follows the advice of the wicked,
> or loiters on the way that sinners take,
> or sits about with scoffers,
> but finds his pleasure in the Law of the Lord,
> and murmers his law day and night.
>
> He is like a tree that is planted
> by water streams,
> yielding its fruit in due season,
> its leaves never fading;
> success attends all he does.
> It is nothing like this with the wicked, nothing like this!
>
> No, these are like chaff
> blown away by the wind.
> The wicked will not stand firm when Judgment comes.
> nor sinners when the virtuous assemble.
> For the Lord takes care of the way the virtuous go,
> but the way of the wicked is doomed.

It was a simple expectation of earthly reward and punishment. The idea of a life after death, or a heaven of reward and a hell of punishment, would not develop for a long time.

Because of this expectation, the Israelite often figured that sickness and pain were the just desert of the sinner, deserved

especially by people who caused trouble for the faithful. For
that reason they would sometimes pray quite sincerely for
disaster to befall their enemies:

> May their own table prove a trap for them,
> and their plentiful supplies a snare!
> may their eyes grow dim, go blind,
> strike their loins with chronic palsy!
>   (Ps. 69:22–23)

On the other hand, it was no surprise for the person who
knew he had sinned against the law to find himself sick. A
psalm describes the plight of such a sinner as he begs
forgiveness:

> No soundness in my flesh now you are angry,
> no health in my bones, because of my sin.
> My guilt is overwhelming me,
> it is too heavy a burden;
> my wounds stink and are festering,
> the result of my folly;
> bowed down, bent double, overcome,
> I go mourning all the day.
>   (Ps. 38:3–6)

This is a lament, but not a complaint. The sinner recognized
his guilt, and accepted the consequences. He only hoped to be
restored, and to prove anew his fidelity to the Law.

It might appear that this view of sickness saw it as the
arbitrary punishment imposed on man by a vengeful God.
Indeed some people look on sickness that way even now. But
there was a deeper insight here—the recognition that sickness
and sin are somehow closely related, and that sickness is a
particularly appropriate result of sin.

It is easier to see why the Israelite recognized the link
between sickness and sin if we are aware that for him, an
external violation of the law was not the fundamental meaning of sin. Such a violation was sinful because it expressed an
attitude that was sin itself: boastful pride. The fundamental
sin was the attempt of a man to build a greatness for himself
without regard for God. The typical example of such pride

was the military conqueror who felt he was invincible, and so
mercilessly and brutally attacked the Israelites. But they read
his fate clearly:

> The Lord God says this:
> Your pride of heart has led you astray,
> who say in your heart,
> "Who will bring me down to the ground?"
> Though you soared like the eagle,
> though you set your nest among the stars,
> I would still fling you down again—
>   it is the Lord who speaks.
>   (Obadiah 1b–4)

No matter how invincible a warrior or how wide his
conquests, God's punishment of sickness and suffering will
humble him.

The teachers of wisdom recognized a clear connection
between a man's pride and his downfall:

> Pride goes before destruction,
> A haughty spirit before a fall.
>   (Proverbs 16:8)

And so those teachers counseled humility as a way to good
health:

> Humble yourself before you fall ill.
>   (Sirach 18:21)

The pride that was the fundamental sin for the Israelite is
quite close to the state of sin as we described it earlier: a
person left to himself, trying to achieve meaning, wholeness,
or value on his own. Such a person might appear on the
surface to be quite successful in his efforts. He might indeed
seem to build a cozy nest among the stars, and gather about
him all the trappings of an earthly paradise. And he can keep
playing that game, that pursuit of a man-made paradise, until
he runs hard into the universal law that all living creatures
suffer and die, and all monuments erode and decay. Sickness
can mean just that: a collision with human limitation, a harsh
reminder of the reality of man's finiteness, his liability to
death. Sickness pricks the balloon of human pride, and

evaporates the illusion that man can get along fine left to himself. The wise Israelite recognized that the wicked man, the proud man, got just the medicine he needed when sickness struck him, and forced him to face his human limits. And so sickness was the sign of sin, the symbol of the true condition of a man left to his own resources, of a man apart from God.

On the other hand, the faithful Israelite acknowledged that he owed his prosperity, his meaning, and his wholeness to God. His prayer, sacrifice, and careful observance of the Law expressed that attitude, and so provided a kind of insurance against needing the lesson taught by sickness: "Humble yourself before you fall ill."

But something went wrong. As the Israelites tried to live according to this view of sickness, with its simple expectation of earthly reward and punishment, they noticed some disturbing inconsistencies. For one, a number of flagrantly wicked people were ignoring God's Law and doing quite well for themselves in the process. The prophet Jeremiah respectfully questioned God about that:

> You have right on your side, Lord,
> when I complain about you.
> But I would like to debate a point of justice with you.
> Why is it that the wicked live so prosperously?
> Why do scoundrels enjoy peace?
> You plant them, they take root,
> and flourish, and even bear fruit.
>
> (Jeremiah 12:1–2)

The question was even more disturbing when the faithful Israelite who asked it was living a noticeably less prosperous life than his wicked neighbor. Then the question became a crisis of faith:

> Look at them: these are the wicked,
> well-off and still getting richer!
>
> After all, why should I keep my own heart pure,
> and wash my hands in innocence,
> if you plague me all day long
> and discipline me every morning?
>
> (Ps. 74:12–14)

The only conclusion that could be drawn if this view of
sickness as God's punishment were true was that something
was radically wrong with God's accounting system!

Another disturbing inconsistency was the shadow of guilt
that sickness cast on a faithful man. If God rewards the
faithful and punishes the unfaithful with sickness, and you
happen to be sick, there is one clear conclusion that people
could draw. You have been secretly unfaithful! You have
committed some hidden sin, but now it is revealed for all by
your illness. Imagine the gossip!

> All who hate me whisper to each other about me,
> reckoning I deserve the misery I suffer.
>
> (Ps. 41:7)

This way of thinking was around even in New Testament
times, and it showed up in Christ's followers as they confronted a blind man. They asked, "Rabbi, who sinned, this
man or his parents, for him to have been born blind?"
(Jn. 9:2)

The book of Job is almost exclusively concerned with this
disturbing inconsistency. Job, an unquestionably just man, is
terribly sick. He asks himself, his friends, and his God, Why
must a just man suffer illness? His friends concluded that,
whether he realized it or not, he must have sinned:

> "A guilty conscience prompts your words." (Job 15:5)

> "Do you presume to maintain that you are in the right,
> to insist on your innocence before God?" (35:2)

> "Avoid any tendency to wrong-doing,
> for such has been the true cause of your trials." (35:21)

But Job persisted in raising this disturbing question, until
he realized something that completely undermined the old
view of sickness as punishment from God, the simple expectation of earthly rewards and punishments. For this expectation
made the relationship between God and man *too* simple. All a
person had to do was observe the Law, and God would be
almost *bound* to make life pleasant for him. This expectation
forgot that God is transcendent, completely beyond the reach

of human powers. It assumed that men could make a legal claim against God—haul God into court in a sort of civil suit!

Because he had this expectation, Job complained to God and in fact asked for a court hearing, with God as defendant! But in the majestic violence of a storm God showed Job his mistake, and confronted him with the truth about his human condition before God. God said:

Who is this obscuring my designs
   with his empty-headed words?
Let me ask you questions, and it is your turn to answer me!

Where were you when I laid the earth's foundations?
   Tell me, since you are so wise!
Have you ever in your life given orders to the morning,
   Or sent the dawn to melt the darkness?
Whose command set down the laws of the heavens,
   and plotted the course of the stars?
Can your voice carry as far as the clouds
   and make the thunder and rain do your bidding?
Who stretches his hand over the cold earth
   to bring forth the buds and blossoms of spring?
Has God's critic thought up an answer?
Or do you really want to accuse me,
   and put me in the wrong to put yourself in the right?
               (Job 38–40 passim)

Job realized the one forgotten thing: he realized *who God is*— and so from what infinite height of freedom God's regard comes. He realized how absurd it was for man to dream he could make demands and accusations against God, to bargain with God, to try to make God obliged to him.

Job responded:

I know that you are all-powerful:
   what you conceive, you can perform.
I am the man who obscured your designs
   with my empty-headed words.
I have been holding forth on matters I cannot understand,
   on marvels beyond me and my knowledge.
I knew you then only by hearsay;
   but now, having seen you with my own eyes,
I retract all I have said,
   and in dust and ashes I repent.
               (Job 42:1–6)

And so Job's question, and with it the whole view of
sickness as a clear and simple punishment for sin, evaporated
like a fog before the warm and brilliant majesty of God. God's
designs are sometimes inscrutable, Job learned. But since God
is faithful, the faithful man must trust in God's love and
accept whatever befalls him.

So the view of sickness changed. No longer was it seen as a
simple punishment. Rather it was part of the mysterious
dealings of God with his people. And as this view changed,
man's awareness of the meaning of his relationship with God
changed, too. No longer was God the guarantor of man's
earthly happiness, a kind of insurance to support man's short-
sighted dreams. God's designs were "beyond me and my
knowledge," and God was working in men's lives to draw his
people gradually to a deeper and purer awareness of him, and
so to a happiness completely beyond their most ambitious
earthly expectations. Fidelity to the Covenant was more now
than observing a law—it was trusting one's life and destiny
into the hands of God.

Now God's people began to regard him as a teacher, a
shepherd to guide them, a father raising well-bred children.
They knew that it was God's steadfast love, his fatherly
compassion, which had preserved the Covenant in spite of
their failures, and had restored his people in spite of defeat
and degradation. Now they saw that this same steadfast love
and compassion were at work in sickness and suffering. Their
response in fidelity meant acceptance of these trials:

> The compassion of the Lord extends to everything that lives,
>   rebuking, correcting, and teaching,
>   bringing them back as a shepherd brings his flock.
> He has compassion on those who accept correction,
>   and who fervently look for judgments.
>   (Sirach 18:13–14)

The valiant woman Judith understood the suffering of her
people as God's fatherly discipline:

> This is not vengeance God exacts against us, but a warning
> inflicted by the Lord on those who are near his heart.
>   (Judith 8:27)

In the same spirit the teachers of wisdom advised their hearers:

> My son, do not scorn correction from the Lord,
>   do not resent his rebuke;
> For the Lord reproves the man he loves
>   as a father checks a well-loved son.
>   (Proverbs 3:11–12)

Suffering and sickness were seen as a sort of initiation into *3.* a special relationship with God. They were like a series of trials through which a person was led by God in order to reach the profound insight into God's designs that was called Wisdom:

> Wisdom brings up her own sons
>   and cares for those who seek her . . .
> If he trusts himself to her he will inherit her . . .
> For though she takes him at first through winding ways,
>   bringing fear and faintness upon him,
> plaguing him with her discipline until she can trust him,
>   and testing him with her ordeals,
> in the end she will lead him back to the straight road,
>   and reveal her secrets to him.
> If he wanders away she will abandon him,
>   and hand him over to his fate.
>   (Sirach 4:11, 16–19)

In a similar way the New Testament Epistle to the Hebrews speaks of sickness and suffering as the training that is the mark of being a true child of God:

> For the Lord trains the ones he loves and punishes all those that he acknowledges as sons. Suffering is part of your training; God is treating you as his sons. Has there ever been any son whose father did not train him? If you were not getting this training, as all of you are, then you would not be sons but bastards.
>   (Hebrews 12:6–8)

In this deeper view, sickness was no longer tinged with fear and guilt, but colored with loving patience and a new kind of expectation. Sickness was the mark of relationship with God, and it bore the promise of God calling a person to a deeper and more pure realization of that relationship. The rewards expected were no longer the easily identifiable riches of the earth; they were the mysterious good things that were to come with the spiritual fullness of God's realm. Suffering was to be accepted in a spirit of patient hope, for it was a way leading close to God.

As the people of Israel and later the followers of Jesus reflected on and lived out this new understanding of sickness, they sought to discern just how sickness was actually to accomplish its task of bringing men closer to God. Two different but complementary interpretations developed, one having to do with he effect of sickness on a person's own attitudes, and the other—quite radical and touching a profound mystery—having to do with the effect of sickness and suffering on the whole people, perhaps on all of history.

The first interpretation saw sickness and suffering as a test and a purification. The writer of the Book of Deuteronomy reflected in this vein on the sufferings of the Jewish people as they wandered through the desert after they had escaped from Egypt. He saw there God testing and teaching:

> Remember how the Lord our God led you for forty years in the wilderness, to humble you, to test you and know your inmost heart—whether you would keep his commandments or not. He humbled you, he made you feel hunger, he fed you with manna which neither you nor your fathers had known, to make you understand that man does not live on bread alone but that man lives on everything that comes from the mouth of the Lord.
>
> (Deuteronomy 8:2–3)

It was the faith of the people that was being tested. Faith, repentance, meant turning away from an attitude of self-sufficiency, where men felt they could get along fine left to themselves, and turning to an attitude of self-surrender, entrusting life and destiny to the hands of God. Of course, if such faith brought tangible rewards, faith would be an easy matter. The kind of measurement of good that is used by men left to themselves would find such faith profitable. Then a person could complacently think he was being faithful and all the while never turn away from the way of thinking and measuring the good that belongs to men left to themselves, the attitude of self-sufficiency that is the root of sin. But when faith in God called for things which contradicted that too-human measure, a person was confronted with a crisis, a painful decision. How far, how radically, would he entrust himself to the hand of God? As the Israelites got their first taste of suffering, many failed the test, and they sent up a cry:

> What good have you done us, bringing us out of Egypt? . . .
> Better to work for the Egyptians than die in the wilderness."
> (Exodus 14:11–12)

Measuring their condition by earthly goods and evils, they failed to understand that God was guiding them, and so failed in the moment of decision. But suffering gradually taught that people to abandon the kind of measurement used by men left to themselves, to rely not on man-made bread but on the call of God.

Such decisions forced confused attitudes to be sorted out, and so probed the inmost heart of a person. Was his trust in God superficial, or did it really reach to the core of his heart?

But, as a good school-teacher knows, a test is not primarily intended to measure a student's knowledge. A test is first of all supposed to *teach*—i.e. to bring a student to discover, develop, and express for himself his own understanding of what he has studied. The test of suffering was not supposed to be a spot check on people's faithfulness to God (what kind of jealously insecure God would need to do that?). The test of suffering was meant to *lead* a person to that deph of faith, to purge out of him the subtle remnants of the state of sin, and so to bring him into a relationship with God that penetrated to his very core, that suffused his entire being. Suffering was meant to purify that relationship from the ambiguities that can prevent a person from fully realizing his meaning, wholeness, and value in relationship with God.

In that way sickness was interpreted as a test and purification of a person's faith. Through sickness and suffering a person could hope to come to a deeper and purer realization of his relationship with God.

But a radical and profound realization dawned with another interpretation of how sickness was to accomplish its task of bringing a whole people, perhaps all men of all time, closer to God.

A small hint of this realization appears at the close of the Book of Job. After Job has suffered catastrophe and sickness, after he has struggled to understand them and finally come to recognize with profound simplicity what it means for a man to stand before God, after he has passed through his ordeal and met his test, his relationship to God has a new character, a kind of priestly character. God instructs Job's misguided friends:

> ... offer a [sacrifice] for yourselves, while Job, my servant, offers prayers for you. I will listen to him with favour and excuse your folly.
>
> (Job 42:8)

Through his suffering Job is in a position to bring God's favor to others and to help to make real God's realm and God's grace in others.

It was the prophet Isaiah who realized that there is a vital connection between suffering and the establishing of God's own realm where suffering and death are overcome, the day for which all Israel had been longing and praying, the day of the Messiah.

The Messiah was supposed to be a glorious king, if he were to establish such a realm. But Isaiah had a different insight:

> See, my servant will prosper,
> he shall be lifted up, exalted, rise to great heights.
>
> As the crowds were appalled on seeing him
> —so disfigured did he look
> that he seemed no longer human—
> so will the crowds be astonished at him,
> and kings stand speechless before him;

for they shall see something never before told
and witness something never heard before:

'Who could believe what we have heard,
and to whom has the power of the Lord been revealed?'
Like a sapling he grew up in front of us,
like a root in arid ground.
Without beauty, without majesty we saw him,
no looks to attract our eyes;
a thing despised and rejected by men,
a man of sorrows and familiar with suffering,
a man to make people screen their faces;
he was despised and we took no account of him.

And yet ours were the sufferings he bore,
ours the sorrows he carried.
But we, we thought of him as someone punished,
struck by God, and brought low.
Yet he was pierced through for our faults,
crushed for our sins.
On him lies a punishment that brings us peace,
and through his wounds we are healed.

(Isaiah 52:13–53:5)

So suffering and sickness, which were the sign of sin and the
symbol of man without God, have become the sign of grace
and the symbol of God's redeeming Messiah. Through suffering will God's relationship with his people be definitively
established, and indeed his relationship with all mankind.

By his suffering shall my servant justify many,
taking their faults on himself.
Hence I will grant whole hordes for his tribute,
he shall divide the spoil with the mighty,
for surrendering himself to death
and letting himself be taken for a sinner,
while he was bearing away the faults of many and praying all
the time for sinners.

(Isaiah 53:11–12)

Jesus Christ was to be that servant:

The Son of Man himself did not come to be served but to
serve, and to give his life as a ransom for many.

(Mark 10:45)

Jesus lived as a faithful and humble Israelite. And he proclaimed the coming of the day for which all Israel had been longing and praying, the establishing of the Kingdom of God. And he faced suffering and death, undeserved as punishment for any sin. But through the complete humiliation of his suffering and death he lifted the burden of the reign of death, of sin, from all men. His resurrection revealed the establishing of a whole new order in which death is finally overcome, and the reign of God is made real—in Jesus Christ himself.

> His state was divine,
> yet he did not cling
> to his equality with God
> but emptied himself
> to assume the condition of a slave,
> and became as men are;
> and being as all men are,
> he was humbler yet,
> even to accepting death,
> death on a cross.
> But God raised him on high
> and gave him the name
> which is above all other names
> so that all beings
> in the heavens, on earth and in the underworld,
> should bend the knee at the name of Jesus
> and that every tongue should acclaim
> Jesus Christ as Lord
> to the glory of God the Father.
>
> (Philippians 2:6–11)

But Jesus' suffering, death and resurrection did not remove sickness and suffering from human life.

It is true that Jesus spent much of his public life healing the sick, and the sick and suffering crowded around him hoping for relief. But there were still sick people left when Jesus had departed from a place. His healing was meant as a sign. Sickness and suffering remained signs of the condition of man without God, signs of the state of sin and the realm of death. Jesus' healing signalled the overthrow of the realm of death and the forgiveness of sin. So when the followers of John the Baptist wanted to know if Jesus was the promised Messiah, it was to his healing of the sick that he pointed:

> "Go back and tell John what you have seen and heard: the blind see again, the lame walk, lepers are cleansed, and the deaf hear . . ."
>
> (Luke 7:22)

But Jesus' primary concern was not healing bodily ills. When the paralyzed man was lowered to him through the roof overhead, it seemed to him that what the man really needed was the firm assurance of his relationship with God: "My friend, your sins are forgiven you" (Luke 5:20). Only afterward, and as a sign and proof of this inner healing, did Jesus cure his paralysis.

What Jesus healed was not so much the particular ailments of the relatively few sick people he encountered, but he healed sickness itself.

For one who follows Christ, sickness is no longer a punishment. It is no longer the unwelcome embrace of the realm of sin and death. It is no longer even a solitary training for spiritual purification. And it is no longer a lonely sacrifice for the good of unknown others.

Christ and those who believe in him form an organic unity, a single reality. In every detail of the Christian's life, Christ is embodied and made real. Through Baptism and Eucharist a Christian participates in Christ. And with Christ and for all who participate in him, suffering and death are linked irrevocably to resurrection and transfiguration: Good Friday is forever one and the same moment as Easter.

For the Christian, therefore, sickness and suffering mean sharing in the very reality of Christ's redemptive suffering. Indeed if anyone desires to follow Christ, it is the cross that he must expect:

> "If anyone wants to be a follower of mine, let him renounce himself and take up his cross every day and follow me. For anyone who loses his life for my sake, that man will save it."
>
> (Luke 9:23–24)

But the cross is Christ's cross—and to bear the burden of the cross is to share in the whole mystery of Christ's redemptive death and resurrection, "sharing his sufferings so as to share in his glory" (Romans 8:17). Such suffering was indeed St. Paul's greatest desire:

> All I want is to know Christ and the power of his resurrection and to share his sufferings by reproducing the pattern of his death. That is the way I can hope to take my place in the resurrection of the dead.
>
> (Philippians 3:10)

To suffer with faith in Christ, abandoning the too-human measure of earthly goods and evils and entrusting oneself into the hands of Christ's father, is to reproduce the pattern of Christ's death. Suffering in that spirit is filled with hope, for it bears the sure promise of resurrection. If we copy Christ's suffering, "he will transfigure these wretched bodies of ours into copies of his glorious body" (Philippians 3:21). The Christian in suffering becomes an imitation and an image of Christ—and "if in union with Christ we have imitated his death, we shall also imitate him in his resurrection" (Romans 6:5).

But there is an even greater significance to sickness and suffering in union with Christ. For to suffer with Christ is also to participate in his work of establishing the realm of God on earth. It is true that God's Kingdom is definitively established by Christ's death and resurrection. But the incorporation of the world as a whole into the reality of Christ is a slow evolutionary process, as is the gradual purification of an individual person. The penetration of God's Kingdom into the whole world makes slow and sometimes ambiguous progress through history, gradually touching and purifying each individual in his relationship with God, gradually incorporating all of humankind and all of history into the reality of Christ. So there remains much work to be done—and it is to be done through sufferings and sickness. St. Paul wrote from a prison cell:

> It makes me happy to suffer for you, as I am suffering now,
> and in my own body to make up all that has still to be
> undergone by Christ for the sake of his body, the Church.
>
> (Colossians 1:24)

For the Christian, suffering and sickness are permeated and
transformed by a clear hope: the expectation of the completion of Christ's Kingdom and his final coming in glory, a glory
that the Christian shares now as a promise, then as fulfillment. For the Christian, therefore, all suffering has the
positive quality of the pains of giving birth:

> You will be sorrowful,
> but your sorrow will turn to joy,
> A woman in childbirth suffers,
> because her time has come;
> but when she has given birth to the child
>   she forgets the suffering
> in her joy that a man has been born into the world.
>
> (John 16:20–21)

All suffering and sickness can be a share in the whole world's
longing for the day of Christ's triumphant return—the glorious fulfillment of the hope of every Christian.

> I think that what we suffer in this life can never be compared
> to the glory, as yet unrevealed, which is waiting for us. The
> whole creation is eagerly waiting for God to reveal his sons.
> . . . Creation still retains the hope of being freed, like us, from
> its slavery to decadence, to enjoy the same freedom and glory
> as the children of God. From the beginning until now the
> entire creation, as we know, has been groaning in one great act
> of giving birth; and not only creation, but all of us who possess
> the first-fruits of the Spirit, we too groan inwardly as we wait
> for our bodies to be set free.
>
> (Romans 8:18–23)

The Christian's hope is for the transformation of the entire
world, the saving, the restoration, the transfiguration of all
men who accept this grace of Christ. And no matter how
agonizing or disfiguring the sickness the Christian suffers, he
can realize that this very suffering helps bring forth the day of
triumph, and his own suffering body will share that triumph:

I will tell you something that has been secret: that we are not all going to die, but we shall all be changed. This will be instantaneous, in the twinkling of an eye, when the last trumpet sounds. It will sound, and the dead will be raised, imperishable, and we shall all be changed as well, because our present perishable nature must put on imperishability, and this mortal nature must put on immortality. When this perishable nature has put on imperishability and this mortal nature has put on immortality, then the words of Scripture will come true: "Death is swallowed up in victory. Death, where is your victory? Death where is your sting?"

(1 Corinthians 15:51–55)

Through sickness and suffering the Christian contributes to the advance of Christ's body toward this day of triumph over the realm of death. Sickness itself has been healed—no longer the sign of defeat by death, it is the mark of Christ's vanguard:

These are the trials by which we triumph, by the power of him who loved us.

(Romans 8:37)

*   *   *

The Christian faith has led us a long way from the attitude implied by the get-well card, where there is no use or value in sickness, and no place for the sick person in the busy pursuit of a plastic paradise.

If we look at the prayers of the Church, an apt alternative to the verses of drug-store consolation cards, we notice two striking attitudes toward the sick.

First is care and concern, for the cross is never an easy thing to bear. The Church therefore prays that God will give strength to the sick and to all who suffer in any way. For instance, the Catholic rites for the anointing of the sick and for the visiting of the sick pray that God will be close to the sick person as a strength and as a healing. They bring to bear Christ's power over the realm of sin and death. In ways like this the Church seeks to strengthen and support the sick person in his time of trial.

The other attitude is one of grateful respect, for the Church recognizes the very great contribution which the sick person makes to the coming of the Kingdom. And so the Church senses that her sick are in a way specially *present* in the congregation, vital participants, though they may be physically absent. They participate intensely in everything that the Eucharist embodies and signifies—the Christian's participation in the saving death and resurrection of Christ.

But there is a problem with looking to religious faith for the significance of sickness. We have tried to discern the pattern formed by apparently disconnected comments here and there in the Bible, and in the process we have gained some idea of the meaning that sickness *should* or *can* have in the Christian faith. That pattern and those ideas, though, are *abstract*, and somehow they sound flat and hollow if they are spoken to a person who really suffers from sickness. That should not be surprising, really—always and everywhere what is really significant in religion is what can't be spoken so clearly. It is a meaning only indirectly expressed by the words of Scripture, a meaning that comes alive unspoken, hidden within the encounter of the believer and the mysteries of his faith.

And so as we continue to seek the significance of sickness, our attention turns to the experience of the sick person himself. We might be surprised to recognize there the quiet and anonymous work of sickness teaching, testing, and challenging, and making real before our dimly perceiving eyes the faint outlines of Christ's death and Resurrection.

Part II
Coping

Sickness means suffering for the sick person, and as well for those who are close to him. The acceptance of this suffering does not come easily, especially when it is death—one's own or another's—which calls for acceptance. But the struggle for acceptance, a spiritual struggle, reveals itself as a teacher of profound and purified faith. And the result of that acceptance can be joy and fruitfulness in suffering.

Chapter 3

There are Depths and Depths

Sickness touches people in a wide variety of forms and a whole spectrum of seriousness and intensity. And so the lived experience of sickness runs a wide range from minor headache and indigestion to terminal cancer. Each depth of sickness has its own particular character, and brings with it a particular kind of challenge. And in each depth of sickness there may hide a particular significance, at least as a possibility or a call.

Common Complaints

The generally healthy person engaged in the business of living in American society—one who is likely to *send* rather than receive a get-well card—is a prime target for a whole battery of common complaints that hardly merit the title "sickness." The energetic salesman pushes himself from appointment to appointment in spite of the congestion of a common cold. The nurse makes her rounds with a smile in spite of a growing headache. The homemaker tends to her hundred tasks in spite of heartburn. But for each it is a bit of a strain, for none is feeling quite "normal."

Common ailments can of course be more demanding, and may become insistent enough to stop a person from doing what they'd like, and so interrupt the business of living. A bad sore throat can pretty well silence the most articulate teacher. A seasoned traveler can be effectively grounded by an attack of diarrhea. And a case of indigestion can kill for a person the liveliest of parties. Then of course the heavier artillery among common complaints—bad colds, mild flu and the like—can wipe out the healthiest person for a day or three.

Most people take these common complaints in stride, and keep about the normal business of living as well as they can. But an interesting pattern appears if we follow to its source the sound of the loudest grumbling about common complaints. Its source is often the energetic, successful person whose involvement in the business of life is quite intense. He doesn't get sick too often, but when he does we hear about it.

For the energetic person, a headache or a cold is a thief stealing his normal abilities and frustrating his efforts and plans. The loud grumbling from this source registers mostly in the "expletives deleted" category. And if the victim is laid up for a day or two, his mind is filled with what he is supposed to be doing, or how far behind in his work he is falling. He feels a kind of outrage, as if sickness had committed a crime against him.

Unspoken beneath his grumbling hides an interesting assumption. A person may be outraged when something he rightfully owns is stolen, but his reaction would be tempered if what is stolen does not really belong to him. Our frustrated victim seems to be assuming that he has undisputed owner-ship of his abilities, and full control over his efforts and plans. He relies absolutely on himself, and considers this unplanned interruption of his usual way of functioning totally unfair. Quietly hiding beneath that assumption is the illusion of the earthly paradise, where everything goes as planned, where the rules are fair, and there are no unpleasant surprises. And the dim shadow of an ancient warrior's boastful pride subtly emerges:

> Though you soared like the eagle,
> though you set your nest among the stars,
> I would still fling you down again—
> it is the Lord who speaks.
>   (Obadiah 4)

A healthy reminder it is, the headache or the cold. Human powers have limits; a man's claim on his life, his efforts and his plans is not quite undisputed. Mild discomforts are subtle notice that there is a claim of eminent domain.

Accidents

A more dramatic challenge is presented by an accidental injury which is disabling for a relatively short time but may require a hospital stay. While the actual interruption of living here may be little longer than for a case of the flu, there is an element of surprise that adds a new meaning to the experience. Most people expect colds, headaches, and occasional bouts with the heavier common complaints. But accidents always happen to the other guy.

A busy homeowner planned to paint all his windows in a single afternoon, and in his hurry he risked leaning from his step-ladder to reach one last corner of a first-floor window. He was surprised at how severe a sprain can result from a four-foot fall. A housewife receiving stitches for a bad gash in her hand will think twice before dropping a sharp knife into the dishwater again. And the office worker daydreaming of warm family and good supper awaiting him as he drove home was shocked to learn that a mechanical failure in a stranger's car could shatter his orderly life in a moment.

The homeowner and the housewife are likely to be quite frustrated by the interruption of their living pattern, but their anger is most often directed at themselves. "Boy, was I ever stupid." Each has become acutely aware how vulnerable are the "normal" routines and patterns of life. Human vulnerability is only too clearly symbolized by his crutches and her bandaged right hand. But both attribute their vulnerability to carelessness. Somehow they know they are responsible for their discomfort, and so they know "it could have been avoided."

Hidden beneath their anger at themselves is the hint that such carelessness is not itself considered part of the genuinely normal human condition, that stupid errors can quite easily be eliminated from one's life. It doesn't take much knowledge of history to realize how unrealistic an assumption that is. Perhaps such a realization lies behind a change that often comes once such homeowners and housewives have vented their anger at themselves. They sometimes come to *laugh* at their foolishness. From anger at what shouldn't be but is, they come to accept the *incongruity* of the human condition: what shouldn't happen very often does, and that's the way it is. This is not the earthly paradise where everything goes as one would wish, and men are not earthly gods who can be expected to do what they should.

But the office worker who is spending a few days in a hospital bed instead of at home to recover from cuts and bruises has a different quality to his surprise. He was minding his own business, and in a moment another car crashed into his life. He knows only too clearly how vulnerable he is, and his aches underline that vulnerability. The homeowner and housewife had a certain comfort: they could see *why* the accident happened and could see a painful but appropriate justice in their suffering. But this man's experience carries the surprise of the irrational, the unjust. And so he may face in a mild way the puzzle that so bothered Job. Why me? What did I do? Where the homeowner and housewife feel anger at themselves and then perhaps a comic acceptance, this man feels only confusion: "I don't understand." And the acceptance to which he is called is deeper. On the surface, of course, his acceptance may seem very simple. "That's the way the ball bounces." But his bruises and above all his painful memory of the shock of unexpected impact reveal beneath that surface, ever so dimly, his meeting with a world that defies any effort to make rational sense of it, a world where justice and order and other human attempts to find a satisfying meaning are themselves only too obviously vulnerable. And as with Job, his question "why me" contains within it a fear that the order of the universe is not entirely reliable. This man is challenged to question the assurances of meaning and happiness which support most people. He could well become cynical and fatalistic. But he could, like Job, come to recognize an assurance of meaning "beyond me and my knowledge," and perhaps he is called to entrust himself not to the only apparently predictable order of things, but to the hands of one who is beyond the predictable and the rational.

A Long Hospital Stay

The accident which leaves a person hospitalized for many weeks and the acute illnesses which requires a long period of treatment or convalescence add several new dimensions to the experience of sickness, each with its own special challenge. Subjection to hospital routine, recurring or continuing pain, and isolation and boredom enter the sick person's life.

Hospital routine

Even a short hospital stay represents a dramatic shift in life style to the patient, but it is experienced as an interruption rather than a change. If the stay extends beyond a few days, though, the change in life style brought about by hospital routine can have a significant effect on a patient's morale and his sense of self respect.

The adult who is accustomed to arranging his own affairs and taking responsibility for others finds himself no longer in control of such things as the time he wakes up, what and when he eats, and in some cases when he can go to the bathroom. He may be accustomed to enjoying a drink before supper, but that may no longer be possible.

He may be in the habit of eating a very large breakfast, and so may even laugh when his morning tray arrives. It may be that his treatment requires a strict regimen, including a carefully regulated diet as well as medication, so that he has little choice regarding what he eats. Even his own body is no longer under his control, but is squeezed, hypodermicked, tested, measured, washed and clothed by others, according to their program rather than his preferences. His capacity for significant choice, for exercising control and responsibility in his own life, is sharply reduced. And with that his sense of self respect dwindles. He may come to feel he is being treated like a thing.

To some extent efforts can be made by the hospital staff to provide for each patient more freedom and control in his own routine. Many hospitals provide menus for meals. More and more nurses habitually try to develop a sort of contract with each patient under their care, arriving at a mutually acceptable daily routine of care that the patient can control, within limits. Care is taken to explain to the patient the nature and purpose of medications and procedures so that he can intelligently and actively cooperate in his care rather than being acted upon like an object.

But very often his sickness itself makes him helpless to care for his most ordinary needs. In effect sickness forces him to relive the helplessness and dependence of a baby. And for an active adult who is proud of his independence, the experience can be embarrassing, or even humiliating.

Humiliation is not necessarily all that bad, of course. There is a salutary irony involved when a self-reliant man is unceremoniously reduced to a common human dependence, and that often before strangers. Such a humiliation challenges the person to a sense of humor about himself: his situation as he is helped with a bedpan bears resemblance to the old Laurel and Hardy routine in which the pompous banker unwittingly loses his pants and struts off down the street. His ability to laugh at himself, though, depends a lot on the depth of his self respect. If his self-image is primarily linked to his achievements and his independence, it will be a long time before he can sense the humor of his situation. But if he realizes that his worth as a person is in his very being, he can afford to laugh, for his humiliation cannot destroy the God-given foundation of his value. Here it is of great importance that those who care for him discover and respect the person that he is, and delicately guide him to accept and value his common humanity and the humor of his situation.

Pain

Pain is one of the most mysterious aspects of sickness. It can vary from a quiet companion always present in the background of consciousness to a violent continuing explosion that fills and seems to burst the mind until the victim is reduced to utter helplessness. Two points along the continuum of pain are of special significance: the threshold, where pain asserts itself in the person's consciousness strongly enough to cause a noticeable response, and the limit of endurance, the point where pain effectively prevents the person from functioning coherently. The pain of one patient may be evident as soon as one is within earshot of his room, but the pain of another might be evident only to the trained eye of the nurse as she observes a subtle tightness of his face. One patient may be able to speak coherently, write a letter or hold a conversation while suffering intense pain, while another may be reduced to helpless cries by comparatively mild suffering.

The factors that govern that variance are many, and some have no direct connection with the type of illness or injury the patient suffers. One's cultural background can make quite a difference in the expression of response to pain. Some cultures encourage outspoken emotions, while others counsel reticence. Some reward expressions of pain with sympathy, while others disapprove such lapses in stoic discipline. Family status can have an effect. The oldest child in a family tends to want to set an example of toughness or discipline, while the baby of the family tends to cry out and expect comforting. A child who feels secure will generally be able to stand more pain than a child who lacks a firm sense of being loved. Further patterns appear in relation to socioeconomic background. Farmers for instance, generally tend to be more stoic. Highly educated people generally tend to expect full relief from medication. (Medical professionals, ironically, tend to be demanding in this regard when they are receiving rather than giving care.)

Attitude has a direct bearing on how much pain a person can bear. Anxiety and anger over the sickness or injury compounds pain, whereas acceptance raises the threshold and the capacity to endure. The person who is confident of recovery tends to withstand pain more easily than one whose hope is shaken or abandoned. A person disturbed by a body-image problem, such as fear that his illness or injury will have a disfiguring effect, expresses a response to pain more often than one who has no such fear. The person who feels isolated from family and friends or from significant human companionship has a harder time coping with pain than one who has been able to keep alive his previous relationships or to establish new ones in the hospital.

Pain can be medically controlled to a great extent. Narcotics can relieve pain, in many cases without necessarily making the patient "dopey." Severe chronic pain can be surgically relieved for relatively long periods. Hypnosis is occasionally used to lock pain out of consciousness. One interesting method for controlling pain is biofeedback training, which enables a patient to develop in himself a meditational state in which he experiences a sense of voluntary control over his feeling of pain. This training is typically given through behavior modification techniques using machines to test brain wave patterns for the "alpha" wave indicative of restful meditation.

Pain, especially intense pain, is more than an interruption of the business of life. Severe pain cuts a person off from his ability even to think, to be aware. His pain becomes his whole world, and all he can hope or pray for is relief, the blessing of sleep, of unconsciousness. There are hints of a particular meaning in pain, though, in the intriguing relationship between pain and acceptance, and the suggestive goal of biofeedback training, a sense of voluntary control over pain. Pain beyond endurance brings tears and the body writhes in one total gesture that shouts "NO!" to the suffering it can't escape. But what if the sufferer said "yes" instead? These hints suggest that acceptance, voluntarily *willing* the inevitable pain, actually reduces felt pain and increases the capacity to endure. But how on earth can a person *want* to suffer pain?

We find here an echo of the experience of Job, whose sufferings wrung many a cry from him until he was brought by God to a full acceptance of his destiny in faith. But such an acceptance is not the easiest thing to come by. Suffering is something most normal people want to avoid as much as possible, and they design their lives to exclude it. But the best-laid schemes often go astray, so men suffer in spite of themselves. Here resignation enters: "grin and bear it," "keep a stiff upper lip." One's desires are in conflict with the reality of his condition, but he endures.

Job went further. He did endure without real complaint, but then he came to see—with some help from on high—that his designs and desires were worthless, empty-headed, before the majestic designs of God. And so he let go of his own plans and more or less blindly abandoned himself to God. Were a person to follow Job, there would be no conflict between his desires and the reality of his condition. For all practical purposes he would have no desires, and the reality would have an unquestioned absoluteness about it. A person would cease struggling against his pain, and find a certain rest in it.

But there is a further step, even beyond the patience of Job. That is to the enthusiasm of Paul, who knew not only *that* God had majestic designs, but knew the design itself,

> the hidden plan he so kindly made in Christ from the
> beginning . . .
> that he would bring everything together under Christ
> as head,
> everything in the heavens and everything on earth.
> (Eph. 1:9–10)

And so Paul not only abandoned himself to suffering, he *embraced* it:

> It makes me happy to suffer for you, as I am suffering
> now,

and in my own body to make up all that has still to be
   undergone
by Christ for the sake of his body, the Church.

(Colossians 1:24)

Suffering here becomes *action* with the profoundest worth.
Pain is no longer interruption and all-pervading frustration, it
is *what one is accomplishing now.* Instead of wracking the
whole person with frustration, it gathers the whole person in a
strenuous act, as if he is concentrating totally on lifting a great
weight. So while the pain is real as ever, the hurt is absorbed,
and the endurance of pain as a negative power against the
sufferer becomes the act of pain as the deed and accomplishment of the sufferer.

A caution is in order, though: Paul spoke out of a long-
established and profound relationship with Christ. He shows
what may be possible, but he respected the physician friend
Luke enough not to bypass normal medical means to ease
pain. It is one thing actively to embrace an unavoidable
suffering, but it is quite another to go out of one's way to seek
pain. Unavoidable pain can bear the mark of God's designs,
whereas selfconsciously sought pain stinks suspiciously of
delusion and self-glorification.

The religious dimension of a human reality, even pain, is an
ambiguous and paradoxical thing.

Isolation and boredom

A person's first reaction to the interruption of living posed
by sickness is usually one of anger and frustration. His mind
tries to keep hold of his customary routine, and his thoughts
are connected with the projects and responsibilities of his
everyday life. His mental life is anywhere but where he is—
sick in a hospital bed. Visitors keep him informed of what is
going on at work, his family visits frequently, and newspapers
give him a sense of being part of what's happening in the
world.

But these links with a wider world weaken as time goes
on, partially because that world grows accustomed to liv-

ing without him, and partially because his own awareness changes and the world he so recently lived in becomes an alien place. Thoughts of the projects and responsibilites of everyday life wither, for he is unable to act upon them. Concerns for his work are set to rest by his less and less frequent visitors, who tell him his colleagues are filling in quite well for him—so telling him unwittingly that he is not really all that indispensable. His family assures him they are managing well, and he senses from the gradually more regulated timing of visits that they have adjusted to a new routine—a routine which includes him only on the periphery. Since he is powerless to act in the world, the daily newspaper passes from being engaging to being entertaining, then to being boring. He looks forward to visitors, but discovers more and more that he has nothing to share—for in his world nothing really happens, and little in their world really relates to him any more.

His experience of time gradually changes. The framework of hours, days and weeks that orders time in the outside world evaporates. One day is like another: Friday afternoon bears no promise of relaxation, and Monday morning no new challenges. Gradually the patient loses any sense of what day it is, for that no longer has any significance. Morning and afternoon are interchangeable. A new time frame emerges, governed by the routine of the hospital. He becomes accustomed to the morning blood pressure check, a light breakfast, the physicians' rounds. Time becomes significant only if it promises something worth looking forward to. Visiting hours . . . and how pervasive the disappointment if no one comes. Meals, especially supper, become the central events of life. Evening is greeted with a sense of pleasure, for it signals the relaxation that leads to sleep.

Activities—reading, handicrafts, writing letters—can fill the void of time to an extent. Reading an absorbing novel, with occasional breaks for naps and meals, can provide a sense of real enjoyment and enrichment. Unfortunately, relatively slight pain can make the concentration needed to read almost impossible, and medication sometimes makes the effort to hold the mind in focus too strenuous. Handicrafts can provide a sense of real usefulness, especially if the sick person has a talent for them. But they have to be useful to somebody else—family, friends, even someone on the hospital staff—if they are to fill the vacuum of time. If patients are able to visit one another, conversation or games of cards, checkers or chess provide a satisfying diversion and a significant form of human companionship. However, patient friendships can have a melancholy quality, for often conversations lack enthusiasm, and deal with past achievements or neutral topics like sports. Sometimes they touch on the medical diagnosis of the patient's illness and have a deceptively objective quality. But the intimate experience of suffering the sickness—and that is the activity in which the person is most closely engaged in the present—does not seem to be considered a thing that can be shared. The patient appears to himself to be doing nothing, or at least nothing he can talk about.

The sinister side of the get-well card has become only too obvious. Its now dusty grin reminds the patient from the bedside table, "Bet you'll be glad to be out of there, and on your own again." The trouble is, the world outside the hospital room has become misty and unreal, and the patient can scarcely imagine any more what it is like to be involved in the business of living a "normal" life. And in the too real world that is now his, there is nothing to do that appears to have any use of value. He is a stranger now to the world his family and friends inhabit. But sadly he is a stranger as well to the world that is now his. He is used to measuring value and sensing meaning in terms of actions, achievements, tangible results, and immediate relationships that are largely on the outside of self. He is a poorly prepared visitor in this world of sickness where most of those values and meanings are absent or irrelevant.

But perhaps something is happening, perhaps he is doing and achieving something or even richer value and meaning that can never be measured in actions and tangible results. And perhaps he is achieving that precisely in his isolation and

his boredom, in a way hidden even from his own consciousness.

The isolation and boredom that grows as a hospital stay
lengthens can call a person to develop spiritually through a
subtle, barely conscious, but profound process.

Most people engaged in the business of everyday living
tend to identify themselves and find their meaning in terms of
their roles, achievements, and immediate interpersonal in-
volvements. Sometimes people even find their meaning and
identity in *things*: a car or a house. But it doesn't take much
analysis to realize that all these things and activities are really
external to one's very self, and in fact can effectively distract a
person, like a mask allowing him to avoid facing himself as he
is. Our culture encourages this sort of flight from what is
within, for it is accustomed to measuring value and meaning
in terms of what is tangible and so external. In fact, the style
of philosophy that is typically American quite readily denies
that the intangible has any reality at all, or at least any
significance worth bothering one's mind about. Such a philosophy needs to encounter sickness.

Sickness gradually weans a person away from roles,
achievements, and most immediate interpersonal involve-
ments. And such a weaning is painful, for gradually a person
is stripped of all the sets and props he has used to act out his
selfhood. The masks are gone, and the hidden being within is
all that remains.

A person faces a challenge at this point, for the being
within is often a stranger. He may well try to hide in whatever
remnants of the tangible world remain. The television remains
on, activities are grabbed at. But a sullenness and a deliberate
strain to avoid boredom marks his effort to flee, and the
tangible aspects of his present role, sickness, are magnified so
that he complains of every pain. On the other hand, he may
allow himself to relax, and let the very quiet being within
gradually occupy his consciousness.

If he does allow his mind to dwell on what is within, an
interesting alteration in his awareness may develop. The

subtle, taken-for-granted aspects of existence rise into clear but unhurried consciousness, and gradually open the sick person's mind to a world of simple wonder that he has forgotten since early childhood. The changing colors of daylight from morning pink to evening gold become intensely clear. The blue of the sky fills the mind, and the progress of a small white cloud across the space defined by the window becomes fascinating. Swirling snow arouses an indescribable pleasure, and the sound of rain or wind a sense of adventure. Incredibly simple things become incredibly significant: the stimulation of a swallow of icewater spreading within one's throat and chest, the exact texture of blanket, sheet and robe, the only too common smell of iodoform. If pain is present, it is no longer a frustration, but it is what the person is doing, in a way an experience interesting in itself. The most obvious things begin to reveal their mystery to the sick person: that the world around him appears to organize itself in relation to his eyes, that his ability to move is dependent on the condition of his body, that his is aware and can direct his awareness by bodily action (moving his eyes) or by inward action (shifting from perceiving to remembering). Dimly and perhaps too deep for speech, he becomes aware of what it means to be a bodily being, yet a conscious being in the world. And he gradually comes to recognize and appreciate the simple being of the things and persons that surround him. In his memory, what he considers important in his life subtly and gradually changes. His actions and achievements recede, and simpler and somehow more human events in his life emerge, moments of sharing, a particularly happy Christmas, the day he met the woman who became his wife. And perhaps a sense of achievement arises on quite a different level: a businessman may recognize the value of his frequent playing with his chidren, a teacher the importance of listening to his students. Gradually, weaned from sets and props and masks, the sick person can come to rest in his own humanity, and find serenity in existence itself.

Perhaps he will go one step further, to recognize that existence is a gift. Then he comes to know that the being within him encounters in itself and in the being of the things and persons around him the quiet presence of the giver of being itself. His serenity then can be touched with joy.

> The compassion of the Lord extends to everything that lives,
> rebuking, correcting and teaching,
> bringing them back as a shepherd brings his flock
> (Sirach 18:13)

Beneath the isolation and boredom that long sickness brings God the teacher can be at work, gradually bringing a person to abandon the kind of measurement of good used by men left to themselves, gradually purging him of the equivocal concerns and ambiguities that can prevent a person from fully realizing his meaning, wholeness and value as a human being in relationship with his God. There can be profound joy in sickness.

A long hospital stay, then, can mean for a person a call to rather profound spiritual growth: to a genuinely humble self-acceptance, to an acceptance and even embrace of God's will even when it conflicts with one's unreflected desire, and to a clarified and purified sense of his human meaning in relation to his God.

Disabling Illness

A challenge yet deeper is faced by the person who receives a diagnosis of debilitating chronic illness like multiple sclerosis. While the person requiring a long hospital stay can look forward with hope for a complete cure, this person knows that complete cure is unlikely, that his disease will affect him for the rest of his life, and may indeed grow progressively worse. The basic challenge he faces in addition to those connected with the other depths of sickness is acceptance: accepting the sickness as a permanent part of himself, confronting the economic consequences of the sickness, and living with the fear of progressive disfigurement or recurring attacks of sickness.

Denial and acceptance

It is no easy matter to accept the diagnosis of an incurable and disabling illness. People often simply don't believe, or apparently don't understand what the doctor tells them, and may ask the nurse or question the doctor again, hoping there is some mistake. Some try to discredit the doctor, and may go to several different doctors as if a person could shop around for a favorable diagnosis the way he would for a used car. But his effort to deny does nothing to change his condition, while money and valuable time for treatment are irretrievably lost.

Less direct forms of denial seek to ignore the illness. A person tries to go about his life as if he had no concern for his health, and he tends to explain away his sickness by referring to it as some relatively inocuous disease. Concern for the future is diligently ignored, and the sick person tries to fill each present moment with intense living. Unfortunately, a by-product of ignoring his disease is often the ignoring of the regimen and precautions that can lessen the seriousness of his condition.

Once a person admits to himself the truth of the diagnosis, the painful challenge remains to accept *himself* as a man sick with a disabling disease. His first response to that challenge may be depression, a feeling that he has no future and that his life is worthless. And that depression can be quite serious, even in some cases tending toward the suicidal. The sick person may refer to himself as a "cripple," and say things like "I don't want to be a cripple the rest of my life."

He is challenged to accept for himself a life that is less than "normal." Especially if he is a young person, though, his self image and life ideal up to now have glowed with apparently limitless possibility. If he is older, he already knows how narrow are the limits within which real lives are lived, and so acceptance may be easier. Nevertheless, he looks at a life ahead with rather severe limits that set him apart from "normal" people. If he rebels at the thought, as if he had a choice in the matter or as if he were being arbitrarily arrested by some sort of secret police, he soon realizes the futility of rebellion. He may become resigned. After all, no one has any ironclad money-back guarantee on the quality of his life. But a bitterness remains in resignation, and that bitterness can have an effect on him more paralyzing and disabling than the disease itself. Granted, his life is not to be as he desired it, and his dreams and ambitions may lie in splinters about his feet. Like Job, he is tempted to curse the day he was born. But desires and dreams, however they may move a man to accomplishment, are not real. The situation he actually faces and what he actually does are the real. He is called to live a real life, not a dream life. So like the man in pain he is called to let go of his plans and desires and abandon himself to the reality of his condition. But more, this sharply limited life is *his* life, his own calling, however different it is from his expectations. If he can come to recognize in the real situation the hidden hand of a provident God, perhaps he can have faith that this, his own life, is to be rich in meaning. With such faith, he may be able actually to embrace his sickness, and to affirm himself not in spite of but *with* his disabling disease. The disabling limits of sickness may then become for him something analogous to the strict limitations placed on an artist by his medium, a fertile framework for creativity and for the expression of rich meaning.

Fears for adequacy

If the sick person can come to accept himself as he is, and have faith in the meaning and value of his own life, he faces fears concerning his adequacy and acceptability in a world that may be less able than he is to see value in his limited life. Will he be able to maintain his place in the world?

Financial problems are only too real. Will he be able to support himself and his family? Will his medical care prove to be an unbearable financial burden? What of his career or career plans? But a deeper concern is meeting the fears and anxieties that fill his mind as he faces an uncertain future, and regaining confidence in himself as a productive person.

His first need will be the courage to try. Efforts at rehabilitation and retraining depend for their effectiveness on the will of the sick person to succeed. But succeed at what? At living a "normal" life, no different from the lives of others? He knows that is unrealistic, though the aim of his efforts could well be described as a life as close to "normal" as possible. Like that of an artist, his success must be estimated within the limits of his condition, but at the same time within its distinct possibilities. His aim is to live *his own* life as well as it can be lived. And so his confidence and his willingness to try will be directly related to the depth of his acceptance. If indeed he can embrace his life as it is, and affirm himself as a person within its limits, he won't lack courage to succeed.

But it may well be that such a successful life will not bring with it economic independence. In a society where self-respect is so closely tied to productivity and "making it on your own," dependence on others, especially on public agencies, tends to bring shame on a person. The assumption prompting that shame in this situation, though, is that there is nothing productive or worthwhile in suffering the limitations caused by sickness. The get-well card strikes again. And so a greater courage is called for: not only to affirm one's own life with its limits, but to do so in the face of an indifferent and perhaps belittling society.

But fears for economic adequacy are only part of the challenge. A much more depressing fear rises when the sick person, considering the strain his sickness places on his family, considering his reduced mobility and the possibility of gradual disfigurement, and considering the social stigma often connected with a disabling illness, wonders whether his loved ones will continue to love and accept him. His fear may be expressed as a concern about being a burden to others. But beneath that concern is a question of his own acceptability. Once again he needs the courage to accept and affirm himself as he is, and the trust that—maybe with a little help to understand—his loved ones will share his affirmation. If he can accept himself and trust his loved ones, his positive attitude may well become a strength to others rather than a burden. Needless to say, those around him have a great responsibility to recognize, accept and respect him as *this person*.

A heavier burden

A disabling disease is indeed a challenge and a test, and it is a test many may fail. Even if the sick person resigns himself to the inevitable, he may be unable actually to embrace and affirm his limited self, and he may be unable confidently to trust the love of others for him. Then an understandable but sad situation can develop. In this case the sick person refers to himself as a "cripple," but his tone does not say "I don't want to be this way," but "Don't make any demands on me." Instead of seeking as much independence as possible, he may emphasize his dependence. In extreme cases, his dependence may practically amount to a reversion to childhood, complete with peevishness and unreasonable demands on those who seek to help him. In this way he is excusing himself from bearing the responsibility to take hold of his own life as fully as he can. Further, he is testing the love of those near him, which he does not fully trust and yet to which he desperately clings. Such a person needs understanding and help—which is nothing to be surprised at, for the challenge he confronts is profoundly difficult.

The lived experience of sickness has many depths, and each depth brings with it a particular kind of challenge and as well the possibility of profound significance. It would be foolish, though, to suggest that the experiences of any two persons are alike, or that anyone can provide a clear set of directions to guide a person in his encounter within his own sickness. Here, as everywhere when the deeper dimensions of human life are in question, what is really significant cannot be clearly and neatly put into words. But words can point to the possibilities that lie in those depths. It is the unique challenge of each person who faces sickness to discover there, quiet and anonymous, the call that is addressed to him personally.

Chapter 4

Dying

A person is called into a depth still more profound if his diagnosis indicates a disease generally considered terminal. The word "cancer," for instance, even in cases when the disease can readily be cured, starkly confronts a person with his own death as a very concrete possibility.

All men die, or so they say. And death is a familiar thing—it fills the newspapers, it enters everyday conversations over the back fence or on the kitchen telephone. But there death is something that happens to others, people we know only remotely if at all. It is one of those things that happens—but not to us.

Awareness of death comes sharper when a loved one dies. Death is no longer remote but very close, and suffering and grief mark the loss it brings. Nevertheless what is felt is the loss caused by death: death itself remains something that has happened to the other person.

It is one of life's most ironic paradoxes that no matter how familiar or how close death may be, it is impossible realistically to imagine one's *own* death. We can dream of being *killed*—and picture to ourselves any number of threatening forces bearing down on us in our helplessness until we just can't look, or until we wake up startled. But the very act of dying itself remains veiled in mystery. No one has the opportunity realistically to rehearse in his imagination his own personal death.

Facing the Fact of Death

The diagnosis of a fatal disease starkly confronts a person with his own personal death. Suddenly death is not a vague termination someday to close a full life, like the last poignant paragraph of a satisfying novel. Death is *now*. It is a concrete immediate possibility *for me*, or perhaps a very real probability, or perhaps even simply a matter of fact in a short time. Death remains veiled in mystery—but now it is a mystery that *I* am entering.

Denial

A person's first response to such a diagnosis is usually shock. He had never dreamed his illness was so serious. Even if he had suspicions, those abstract and remote thoughts suddenly become real and very present. Yes, it is *me*—*I* am being called to confront death.

Such a shock is by no means easy to bear, and if a person is told of his condition without being prepared, starkly and without compassion, the news can provoke an emotional upheaval that might actually hasten death. For that reason most physicians are extremely cautious in informing a patient of a fatal diagnosis, and many prefer simply to leave the patient in ignorance. This latter course though leads to other problems.

If the sick person is fortunate enough to be informed frankly and compassionately of his condition, his first thought may be that there must be some mistake. After all, he feels only a little tired, a little run down. He questions his physician, perhaps asking him to have another doctor corroborate his opinion. He may even accuse his physician of incompetence and turn to another, or to a series of others until he finds one who will let him deny his true condition.

Another person may calmly accept the diagnosis, but then speak of his illness as some other disease that is much less threatening. Or perhaps he will accept the disease but simply fail to face its implications: he will speak of the time when he will return to his work, of his plans to travel upon recovery, or of things he hopes to accomplish when he feels better.

We are so used to living in terms of the future that plans, hopes and expectations form the major motif of consciousness. But the obvious implication of a fatal illness is that for this person is no future, or at least a very short one. Plans, hopes and expectations expressed by a dying person are poignantly ironic. Sometimes he may recognize that and laugh at his own foolishness. But looking to the future is a habit of awareness that·is hard to erase, especially since dying—coming to that point when there is no future of the sort we are accustomed to—is something beyond a person's imagining. So from his amusement at the incongruity of his thoughts the sick person may turn to an alarmed silence, for what thoughts *are* appropriate? Despite the conscious acceptance of his diagnosis, a person's mind plays tricks on him and clings to the familiar world he must soon leave. Mind and emotions shy away from the mystery of dying.

It may well be that a person is not informed of his condition. He entered the hospital for tests, or for an operation of an ostensibly routine kind. And he knows nothing—or he is given misleading information. As time goes on, he wonders why he notices no improvement, or why he is given no projected time he may return to normal life. He wonders why the physicians' visits are so routine—or so infrequent. He senses a lack of ease on the part of the nurses. And so he may ask her, "am I sicker than I think I am?" Her embarrassed, ambiguous response only compounds his suspicion. He may have enough knowledge of his disease to recognize its symptoms himself. "Do I have cancer?" And physician or nurse either confirms his suspicion or denies it a bit too vehemently. In either case his trust in those who care for him undermined, for at least until now they have concealed the truth, and perhaps they continue to do so.

Such suspicion can poison the sick person's relationship with those who care for him. He senses a conspiracy of denial, and begins to mistrust everything he is told. Impatience and bitterness tinge and then pervade his dealings with the hospital staff, and begin to color his relationship with other persons as well. The tragic result of this poison is that the dying person becomes more and more alienated from those around him, left to face death alone and without the support of persons he can trust. The terror of his confrontation with death is compounded.

But sometimes the effort to conceal the truth leads to situations that are almost comical. One patient, though he was not told his condition, was quite certain he was dying. He noticed the efforts of his wife and of the hospital staff to avoid certain topics of conversation, and assumed they would be hurt to know the truth. They in turn feared such knowledge would cause him to become seriously depressed. Their little game of let's pretend continued until the patient confided his concern for his wife's feelings to a hospital staff member, who assured him his wife knew all along. Touched and amused by one another's concern, husband and wife then quite calmly worked together to put his affairs in order in the little time that remained.

The way each person walks to confront his own dying is as unique to him as the habits, games, and little foibles by which he coped with living. One patient was fully informed and understood his condition completely, but he would never use the words "death" or "dying". Another was told nothing but knew full well his condition, his physician and nurse knew he knew, and he knew they knew he knew. But they played a genial game of let's pretend until the end. Another would speak of the future and describe his illness as some minor ailment to everyone but one nurse in whom he confided his wrestling with the truth.

The path to acceptance

Facing the fact of a fatal diagnosis is a long way from fully accepting death. For most people it is just the first step in a difficult and sometimes bitter journey.

A person may accept his diagnosis and recognize that it is

now he that is called to confront death. But an insidious question, a very natural question, may pop into his mind. Why? Why *me*, of all the people in the world? This question is more likely the younger and more active a person is, the more promise the future seemed to hold for him. It seems unjust that he should die, cut short from the full life he expected. Death, after all, is acceptable only as the termination of a full and happy life. It makes no sense that it comes *now*—there is too much left to accomplish, too many responsibilities to be met, too many needs to be filled. Why me? What have I done to deserve such a fate?

It is a natural question. But beneath it lies one or another assumption about life—assumptions that have by no means been proven true. One is that every person is entitled to a full and happy life. It is this assumption that allows our culture to distinguish between a happy death, dying in the fullness of years touched by happy memories and surrounded by loved ones, and a tragic death, the lonely death of a younger person of promise, or the parent of young children. However different the consequences of death may be for those who remain behind, death itself does not appear to make such a distinction, nor to recognize any title to a "normal" life expectancy. The other assumption is that death follows some order of justice, or is a punishment for evil ways. This idea lay behind the painful confusion of Job, who suffered so in spite of his goodness that he came to question the justice of God himself. Indeed it sometimes happens that a person will respond to a fatal diagnosis with anger at God, or at least with a question like Job's. The question is a natural one—why me? And there is no direct answer to it. There is only the response Job received from the awesome majesty of God and the simple recognition that God's thoughts are not like the thoughts of men.

The more sophisticated person may be consciously aware that it is useless to question his fate, and terribly naive to pout at God. So he takes his stand in stoic resignation. But those quite natural feelings remain, only now seek an outlet in disguised ways. The patient will not question fate, but may find many opportunities to question the competence or effectiveness of the hospital staff. He vents no rage at God, but bristles with impatience at his nurse. The root of his impatience is the same very natural question, but in its disguises it is more difficult to deal with. So this step along with the path to acceptance may be a bitter one for the dying person and as well for those around him.

Sometimes a dying person may play the game children often play at bedtime. Daddy, may we just watch this one TV program? May we play just one more game of cards? May we have milk and cookies first and then go to bed? One person may beg to live to see a son graduate from college, another to see her married daughter's baby born. Before that, death would be unacceptable, but after that . . . Of course, if the person does live to see what he desired to, he is likely to find another cause for postponement. Indeed he may have accepted that there is no guarantee or title to a full life, but he tries to get his full life piecemeal, all the while viewing death as the vague termination that comes *after* all is accomplished, rather than as the insistent mystery that confronts him *now*.

A person may respond to a fatal diagnosis without bitterness and without childish attempts at postponement, but in a way that is a bit unnerving. One patient was gently told that her sickness was a fatal one, and she simply turned toward the wall and remained silent, waiting passively for death to come. All connection with the world in which she still lived was severed, and her only apparent action was to wait. She was to endure death, so she would endure in silence.

By contrast, many dying persons express a genuine joy in their condition, perhaps much like the joy in long illness described in the preceding chapter. Sometimes that positive acceptance is expressed in terms of a religious faith in immortality, sometimes in terms of an appreciation for the goodness of life as the person has lived it. Sometimes again it is expressed indirectly by the spirit or manner of a person as he continues to interact with others and to occupy himself with present concerns—a letter, a game, a book.

The difference between these two responses to impending

death suggest quite different attitudes. The woman who waited in silence portrayed an attitude of resignation—the refusal to fight any longer. With such an attitude a person remains utterly passive, and death is something that happens to him, a catastrophe that strikes him. The other persons portray an attitude of active acceptance. Here death is no longer simply a blind catastrophic force: it is something one actively meets. Perhaps dying is seen as an act which a person is called to achieve, perhaps as a final challenge and even adventure.

Acceptance in the face of one's own death is an attitude that is partly unique and incommunicable, the utterly personal meeting with the unimaginable. Probing that aspect of dying will lead us into mystery, where we can form only intimations and guesses of its significance. But acceptance is also partly a matter of the relationship the dying person has with the people around him, with the world he is about to leave behind.

The Process of Dying

Except in cases of accidental death or an acute fatal illness like a sudden heart attack, dying does not appear as a moment of trauma, but as a gradual process. Part of the process is walking the path to acceptance. Another significant part is the dying person's changing relationship to the world in which he has lived and to the persons with whom he lives.

Letting go of that world is a painful process, especially because a person leaves it to go into the unknown. Unfortunately the pain and distress of the process may be compounded by failures in his relationship with others.

The dying person and his world

A dying patient may discover that the doctor's visits become less and less frequent as death approaches, and that nurses spend very little time with him. He knows they are busy, and must devote their time to patients they have hope to heal. But he senses—now that he is dying—he is not of much importance to them. Sometimes even his family and friends visit less and less frequently, or when they do visit have very little to say. He begins to feel useless, abandoned by his world before he is ready to let it go. The assumption beneath the get-well card becomes especially cruel.

A serious factor in his relationships is *truth*. Genuine communication with others presumes an open acceptance of the person's real situation—that is, he is dying. And whether or not he has been told, he most probably knows it. If those with whom he might speak persist in pretending, denying his situation, nothing more can be communicated than polite nothings. In the midst of chatter the dying person remains painfully alone with the one thing that really concerns him, and he does not know where to turn for support.

But a dying person is not dead. This world is still his home, and he may be able to enjoy it with a simplicity and sensitivity he has never known before. For the dying person each living moment can be precious—not that he clings to it, but that he recognizes and appreciates its value. Even simple chatter, once grounded in an open awareness of the truth, can be an intense pleasure. The dying person wants to live each present moment fully as he can, to continue living in his world until he himself is ready gradually to sever the ties, gradually to close his relationships.

Little things can be very important. Especially if a person has had a long stay in the hospital, the room he has occupied is now familiar, and one or another nurse may have become a friend. Changes of room, of nurse, or of routine can have the effect of tearing a person out of his familiar world. The adjustment which another person might take easily in stride becomes disturbing to a dying person, for such change complicates the already very demanding process of adjustment and acceptance he is going through. The dying person needs to have a familiar home in this world until he is ready to relinquish it.

The most common image of a happy death is that of dying

at home, surrounded by loved ones and sharing to the end their familiar life. It is not always possible or even advisable for a person to die at home. But when and where he can be at home, the process of his dying can be filled with the awareness that people he cares most for accept him and will share with him this time that is most trying and most significant. He has the opportunity to savor the world most familiar to him, and to take his leave gently and gradually from the surroundings in which he lived. He is free from the sometimes businesslike routine of a hospital, and allowed to set his own pace in this precious time.

Letting go

At least in relation to this familiar world, dying is a gradual process of disengagement, of letting go. One by one good-byes are made—sometimes in so many words, sometimes in an everyday visit or conversation in which an unspoken understanding passes. Gradually the person's interest in the everyday affairs of the family and friends wanes, and he is found more and more frequently in silent thought, even contemplation. His attention turns away from a world that is more and more a thing of the past for him.

However, the person who cannot accept death may cling to his familiar world. He demands more and more attention from those around him, sometimes pestering them for incidental services, sometimes begging just not to be left alone. He may begin to demand assurances of their continuing love and care, perhaps even accuse his family of failing to love him. He insists on as much control over his surroundings as possible, perhaps demanding that things be arranged in a certain way, or that particular keepsakes be left close to him.

Such an effort to cling to the familiar is readily understandable, for the dying person senses that the only world he knows is gradually slipping away from him, leaving him to confront a terrifying unknown. He cannot stand to be left alone with his fears, especially with the nameless fear of the unimaginable confrontation with death itself. And so he clings to what he can manage, to what is familiar to him.

The gradual detachment from the world that marks the path of acceptance reveals a different spirit. Far from rejecting his loved ones, he remains close to them to the end—yet more and more that closeness remains unspoken, and fewer everyday concerns are shared. Care is received with simple appreciation, and the dying person is himself careful not to make unnecessary demands. He appreciates the moments he has to enjoy life, but relinquishes claims or hopes for a future. He suffers pain, but not trauma. He knows fear—for fear is only reasonable before the unimaginable. But terror does not strike him. Quietly he turns from what is behind him to the unknown he faces.

It is not that difficult to see how letting go of this world is appropriate for a dying person, even if all we know of death is the death of others. After all, we are part of the world the dying person leaves. We feel a profound loss when a loved one dies, and we can assume that dying implies a corresponding separation for him. And everything that may have been important to him is rather obviously torn from his possession. Any wealth he had is transferred to others, his family lives on and gradually grows quite accustomed to life without him. His achievements now benefit others, if time does not completely swallow them.

Indeed, a very evident lesson learned from the death of others is that we have here no lasting home. So clear is that lesson that efforts to build an earthly paradise, once recognized as such, are obvious illusions. From this point of view the person with a terminal illness is not so different from anyone else. So a comedian could declare he had a terminal illness: life. And another defined "fatal illness" as "a period of suffering inevitably ending in death," and facetiously used the same definition for "life." To live is to be subject to death, not as a vague termination someday to close a full life, but as an ever-present possibility. Any moment may be the *now* when I am called to let go, to yield my hold on everything that has made a familiar world for me. And if in living a person maintains that quiet recognition that this is no lasting home, then in dying the letting go is not likely to be traumatic.

Indeed, for anyone who takes seriously the law that all living creatures suffer and die, the diagnosis of fatal illness merely confirms what he understood all along, and gives it a definite now.

But it is one thing to turn away from the familiar world, and it is quite another to confront the mystery of dying.

Probing the Mystery

The very act of dying is beyond the reach of the imagination. And needless to say it has never been accurately described to us by someone who has been through it. What we directly know of dying is precisely nothing. Death remains veiled in mystery.

Probing that mystery is bound to be a fruitless effort, if we expect to arrive at some definite knowledge of death. Death will always be the archetype of the unknown. And yet we can talk with some amount of sense because there are hints and suggestions that point into its mystery in the knowledge we have of death of others, in any close brushes with death we may have experienced, and in some ideas about death contained in the Christian tradition. The effort to probe the mystery is a little bit like putting together a jigsaw puzzle: fitting together the pieces we know can help us guess the shape of the missing pieces. But all we can hope for is a guess, an intimation. Death remains veiled in mystery.

Going from what we know

Perhaps the aspect of the death of others that is most significant here is the variety of responses to the approach of death. One will deny his condition, totally unable to face the fact of death. Another will be angry at its unjustice. For one death is a tragic interruption of a promising life, for another it is a satisfying conclusion. One will be filled with terror at death's approach, while another may welcome death with relief and gratitude. One clings to the world he must leave, desperately fighting off the inevitable separation. Another serenely takes his leave as a courteous guest might bid good-bye. Each is different, yet each truly reflects an aspect of death.

Our reaction to a death we may have witnessed tells us more. This person was present with us a moment ago, talking with us and looking at us. Then suddenly he is not there, and just a shell remains. We are struck with a sense of mystery. And perhaps we feel shock or even horror. If death comes suddenly or with violence, especially to someone we love, the shock and pain is intense. Suddenly he is gone, torn away and destroyed. Death reveals itself as destruction, ruin and devastation, and in the face of it a person is utterly helpless.

As we piece together what we know of the death of others, the shape that emerges is by no means clear. Death is the terrifying unknown, the archetype of injustice and absurdity. It is a satisfying conclusion. It means painful separation; it means a leave-taking. It is helplessness in the face of ruin and devastation; it is welcome relief. Dying is all these things at once: promising yet threatening, terror yet peace, destruction yet completion. But just how these contradictory aspects of death fit themselves together is not clear, doubtless not even to the dying person himself. Perhaps this very uncertainty and ambiguity is a hint of the shape of death's mystery.

We can find further hints about the act of dying from our own close brushes with death. There does seem to be something to the idea that our whole life passes before our eyes in an instant. Perhaps it is not like a sped-up movie of every single event of our past, but a lot of people have had the experience of their life gathering itself together as a whole into this one moment, in a single flash of recognition. It is as if we see ourselves in a mirror and recognize ourselves all at once, and say yes, this is me.

A common dream that is symbolic of death gives another hint about that missing puzzle piece. Many people dream that they are losing their balance and are about to fall, usually into a dark chasm. At that moment they jerk awake, grabbing hold of the bed and kicking the blankets every which way.

The experience is one of losing balance, and then reaching out for support. It might not be too much of a guess to suppose that if we were actually dying we would claw out and find nothing to grab hold of. It would be like falling alone down into that dark chasm with all our familiar supports gone from us.

A girl who was hit by a car later described the feelings she had at that moment. She said to herself, well, things are out of my hands now. She felt kind of relief, and at the same time something like curiosity about what was coming. She said it was like being in a roller-coaster: the thing roared and swerved according to its own rules, and the only thing to do was to trust it and hang on.

Hints from the Christian tradition

Nowhere in the Bible or in the Christian tradition is there a clear description of the act of dying. Death has a very significant place in the New Testament, especially the death of Jesus. But his death is described from the outside—again the death of another. And much is said of what is to come after death—but that is expressed almost exclusively in ambiguous symbols. The most unambiguous statement about heaven, for instance, is also the least enlightening: St. Paul says of himself, ". . . this same person was caught up into paradise and heard things which must not and cannot be put into human language." (2 Cor. 12:3–4). Still there are hints that suggest a definite shape and significance in the act of dying.

One hint is in the idea that after death comes the judgment, the final and unalterable determining of a person's eternal destiny. Judgment is a simple enough idea if we are considering a saint or a villain of unmitigated malice. Here the moral condition of a person is clear, and judgment is simply the final closing of a clear case. But the moral condition of most people is ambiguous at any given moment of life, neither unquestionably good nor inexcusably bad. Here the naive image of an account book or a scale is sometimes used to express the manner of judgment, but both images do real harm to one's understanding of Christianity. They turn one's goodness before God into a quantifiable thing, turn the awaiting of judgment into something like an IRS tax audit, turn salvation into something like net worth instead of grace, and turn God into a glorified accountant. Ambiguity is better than such images.

Several aspects of judgment may shed some light on the mystery of dying. One is the very ambiguity we have noted in any person's moral or spiritual condition at any given time. Another is the recognition that what is at stake in judgment is not conventional moral uprightness of the sort that makes a person acceptable in respectable society, but one's justice before God, which is a matter of living out the relationship with God that is freely given as grace in Christ. One's moral behavior is significant only as the lived expression of the life of grace. The third significant aspect of judgment is its finality: whatever the ambiguity of one's life, his stance in relation to God becomes final and unalterable after death. And the whole of one's life is gathered into that final stance— so that judgment is not only a decisive moment; it would seem to be a moment of *decision* in which the person as a whole is engaged.

A second hint may be discerned in the Catholic doctrine of Purgatory. This doctrine serves as an attempt to reconcile the ambiguity of a person's moral or spiritual condition with the utter purity appropriate for those who dwell directly in the presence of God. But it adds to our pondering one very significant notion, that however final and decisive the moment of death may be, there is place for a kind of growth or purification on the other side of the act of dying. The last act of a dying person then may well not be his "last breath," his last action in the world he has shared with the living. His final act in the sense of completion may be his entry into the mystery of death. Perhaps, then, the dying person—while from all appearances be his passive before death—is really doing something profoundly active and decisive. Perhaps it is indeed appropriate to call dying an *act*.

We learn that after judgment the everlasting destiny of a person is to dwell in heaven or hell. The New Testament has much to say about heaven, most of it of course expressed in ambiguous symbols. Regarding hell, apart from a few references to a burning garbage dump and the gnashing of teeth, the Bible chooses to leave the specifics to the imagination of a certain kind of preacher. Perhaps the key to the biblical description of heaven is that the faithful will share the triumph of the risen Christ: ". . . from heaven comes the savior we are waiting for, the Lord Jesus Christ, and he will transfigure these wretched bodies of ours into copies of his glorious body. He will do that by the same power with which he can subdue the whole universe." (Phil. 3:20–21). "When this perishable nature has put on imperishability, and when this mortal nature has put on immortality, then the words of scripture will come true: Death is swallowed up in victory. Death, where is your victory? Death, where is your sting?" (1 Cor. 15:54–55). The faithful will have an everlasting home, "a house built by God for us." (2 Cor. 5:1). Heaven is presented as a place where the faithful will rejoice to dwell with their Father, and he will comfort them: "'Here God lives among men. . . . He will wipe away all tears from their eyes; there will be no more death, and no more mourning or sadness. The world of the past has gone.' Then the One sitting on the throne spoke: 'Now I am making the whole of creation new.' he said. (Rev. 21:3–4).

A further dimension of the promise of heaven was expressed by the Second Vatican Council. Not only will heaven present the faithful with the ever-new joy of dwelling with God, but it will also restore what they have loved and tried to accomplish during their lives, and perhaps lost to death and decay. "After we have obeyed the Lord, and in His spirit nurtured on earth the values of human dignity, brotherhood and freedom, and indeed all the good fruits of our nature and enterprise, we will find them again, but freed of stain, burnished and transfigured." (Church in the Modern World, #39). The doctrine of heaven shows that death can indeed be a moment of complete fulfillment: fulfillment of what we have worked for and loved in life, and fulfillment of our deepest longing for union with God.

Such a hope for heaven may fill a dying person with confidence and joyous expectation. But there is an insidious danger in hopes for immortality. It can easily happen that a person may use such hopes as a way to deny the reality of death. He will not die—he is only going for a short trip to a new and beautiful home. His mistake is twofold. First, he fails to recognize the reality of death. Second, he fails to recognize the promise of heaven for what it is: a promise, not a fact.

A too-easy belief in immortality fails to face the fact of death as utterly unknown, as an unimaginable mystery. Only a fool would advance toward death as if he knew all about it, as if he had everything under control. Often a person who has expressed a serene acceptance of death because of his faith is struck by a radical doubt at the last, for after all he has no real evidence for his belief, and it has come to him not as fact but hardly distinguishable from hearsay. And so his confidence collapses in panic as he recognizes that for him too death is mystery.

Further, the Christian tradition is quite clear in emphasizing that everything that is revealed about heaven and immortality has the character of a promise and a hope, not of a foregone conclusion. It would be a terrible mistake—indeed it would be the mistake of the Pharisees of the New Testament—to take heaven for granted, as if a person had title and key and needed only make the short trip through death to take possession of it. As far as we can know on our own, and as far as we can count on as under our own control, death is destruction, devastation, ruin and darkness—with perhaps a bit of confused and ambiguous hope thrown in. Heaven is something we don't know about on our own, something that is not under our own control. Heaven is revealed as the promise of God, and it is offered as a gift of God that he gives out of his complete freedom. He owes a person nothing. Hence in dying a person can only hope in

God and rely on him and his promises, not on himself. A
significant insight into death is suggested by the fact that the
scriptures and tradition emphasize strongly that death is the
result and the symbol of sin, in particular of Adam's sin. Sin
separated man from God: man decided to go it alone. Death
is where that decision leads, for man is helpless alone and
crumbles into nothing. And so the destruction, the devastation, the ruin, the falling into darkness that is part of death is
a dramatic manifestation of what sin means.

But when Christ definitively established the realm of God
and so founded once and for all the stable relationship
between God and men, he would also have radically changed
the meaning of death. How significant it is that the realm of
God is established precisely through Christ's *death*, a death
which led to resurrection. But that means as well that the
person who believes in Christ should experience death differ-
ently, for he understands his own dying as a participation in
Christ's act of dying.

Just how *is* the death of a believer different?

That question pokes directly into the center of the mystery
of dying, and indeed brings us into the mystery that is at the
center of Christianity: Christ's own act of dying and the
reason why his death led to the resurrection. Here, too, death
remains veiled, and we know only the sketchy description of
Christ's dying given in the Gospels, and theological reflections
on its meaning which are themselves somewhat ambiguous.
But we can try to piece together the puzzle.

The first and perhaps most important point is that Jesus
died a fully human death. That means that he suffered the
same fear, loneliness, destruction and darkness that is so
much a part of human death. In fact, he seemed to have
suffered it more intensely than anyone else: "and a sudden
fear came over him, and great distress. And he said to them,
'My soul is sorrowful to the point of death. Wait here, and
keep awake.' And going on a little further he threw himself on
he ground and prayed that, if it were possible, this hour might
pass him by." (Mk. 14:33–35). Luke records that "his sweat

fell to the ground like great drops of blood." (Lk. 22:44). The depth of Jesus' loneliness and emptiness in the face of death is embodied in that anguished cry of abandonment "My God, my God, why have you deserted me?" (Mk. 15:34). The horror and fear of dying was apparently very much a part of Jesus' act of dying.

But another element is equally apparent in Jesus' dying. When he prayed in the Garden of Olives, his anguish was matched by his dedication to his Father: "But let it be as you, not I, would have it." (Mk. 14:36). And according to Luke, his words just before the moment of dying were, "Father, into your hands I commit my spirit." (Lk. 23:49). Jesus' act of dying appears then to be an act of giving himself completely over into the hands of the Father.

St. Paul says that this ultimate obedience to the Father, this complete giving of himself into the Father's hands is the reason why Jesus' death led to the resurrection. "Christ became obedient for us unto death, even to death on a cross. Therefore, God also has exalted him, and has given him the name that is above every name." (Phil. 2:8–9). When we realize that Jesus' obedience led him right into the horror and fear that we saw in the Garden of Olives, right into the destruction, ruin, loneliness and darkness that are so much a part of death, we can see how radical and complete was the trust and confidence in the Father that was embodied in his act of dying. Jesus placed himself totally into the hand of the Father, and the hand of the Father raised Jesus from the dead.

Now that we have assembled all the pieces that we have of our puzzle, perhaps we can start filling in a few of the outlines of that mysterious missing piece, the act of dying.

The first thing we can guess about the missing piece of the puzzle is that death really is an act, and not just something that happens to us that we can do nothing about. If dying is the decisive moment for our eternal destiny, then it seems sensible to suppose that there is some decision made by a person in dying. Further, we have seen that death is ambiguous: there are many loose ends left dangling as a person faces death. For instance, his life is a mixture of good and bad. His state of mind is a mixture of readiness and fear. Somehow in the very act of dying all these loose ends have to be gathered into a decisive knot, into that yes or no to God. Hence there is reason to say that there is some kind of final decision made in the very act of dying. What looks to us like a passive suffering could well be a profoundly active decision.

And yet that decision would not be just one more act, isolated somehow from the rest of life. This one decision would have to be the focus and the tying together of all that has gone before. Perhaps that experience of seeing our whole life gathering into one before our eyes, that we may have in a close brush with death, is a part of this gathering of our whole life into one final decision.

But what is the nature of this decision that seems to be at the core of the act of dying? What has to be decided? What would make a right or a wrong decision? To make our educated guess about this question, we need to look again at what the dying person apparently experiences.

The impressions we can gather from the death of others, from our own close brushes with death, and even from what our faith reveals about death adds up to an obscurity and an ambiguity. Death appears as a completion, as a relief, as leading to the promise of heavenly fulfillment. At the same time, and even more intensely, death appears as a violent interruption, as separation and loneliness, as helplessness, as falling into darkness. The important thing here is that the ambiguity of death makes the dying man uncertain: he does not know for sure what death has in store for him. His destiny is very definitely out of his own hands. A man discovers his ultimate helplessness as he comes to die: he comes to the farthest limit of his own being, and finds it is not enough to save him from destruction and darkness. Death throws a man beyond what he can know and predict and control—it is very much like that dream of falling into the dark chasm, only there is nothing to grab hold of. To die is to be forced to let go of everything and to let oneself fall, out of control. The act of letting go seems to be at the heart of the mystery of the act of dying.

Where is the decision in this act of letting go? Wouldn't we be almost forced to let go of ourselves? The decision is not to let go or not; it is rather what we let ourselves go *into*. What are the possibilities? First, the person could say to himself that there is nothing to fall into. The chasm is dark: what death holds is obscure and ambiguous. If the person would despair of anything beyond what he could know and control, he would see simply darkness, and let himself go into darkness. For him, dying would seem to mean falling alone into that dark chasm.

Or perhaps the person thinks he has the title and key to his heavenly fulfillment—in one form or another. He thinks he needn't let go of his destiny at all: his future is assured (we might call this presumption). For him the act of dying will be a shock, for what he thinks he grasps will be torn from his fingers, and he too will hurtle alone into the chasm. "Anyone who finds his life will lost it." (Mt. 10:39).

But there remains the possibility of trust. We know we cannot overcome the destruction and darkness of death by ourselves. And yet we know there is One who can. And we know of the promise of heavenly fulfillment that God has made to us. Only at this decisive moment, we realize that God is a just judge as well as a merciful father. He is indeed free, and we have no guarantee that he will choose to grant us what he has promised. God is no servant of ours: he owes us nothing. Then dying would seem to be the letting oneself fall into the hands of God, ready to accept whatever he wills for us. Perhaps we can say it is like letting oneself fall into that dark chasm, only not alone: trusting rather that God's hands will catch and hold us. It is like trusting that roller-coaster. Then our dying word, our final decision, would be, "Father, into thy hands I commit my spirit." And that decision would put us into company with Christ in his own act of dying. It would mean placing ourselves with Christ into the hands of the Father, hoping in the power and mercy revealed in Christ. To die in this way would be to die with Christ.

This interpretation of the mystery of dying is at best an educated guess, an intimation. If it is correct, it reveals a profound connection linking death with the central mystery of Christianity. Indeed the attitude with which a person faces death appears to correspond quite closely with the attitude of faith which accepts the free gift of grace, as opposed to the attitude of sin which chooses to stand alone in the attempt to have things always under one's own control.

It is possible to see in this regard how it is the inner attitude of daily living that becomes focused and knotted into the final decisive act of dying. The person who must always be in control, who must always be sure of himself, may find dying a terror and a trauma. On the other hand, a person who has a sense of humor and detachment about his own security, who can meet the unpredictable demands of life with creative acceptance may well find when he comes to die that he has been dying with Christ all his life.

The death of others is a familiar thing, and death is as ordinary occurrence as a graduation or a wedding. It is something that happens in life, a common thing as it happens to others.

But *my* graduation is special, and my wedding is a unique and wonderful experience—for now it is I who don cap, gown and hood, or it is I who walk in beauty down the aisle. So familiar from the outside, these common rites of passage suddenly become unique, for it is I who perform the familiar ritual.

The day comes when it is my turn to walk with death, and to enter the unique mystery of this familiar ritual.

I have no opportunity to rehearse.

And yet hopefully I have been rehearsing for this moment throughout my life. The instructions for the ritual are very simple and very succinct. So we are advised:

> In your minds you must be the same as Christ Jesus:
> His state was divine,
> yet he did not cling
> to his equality with God

but emptied himself
to assume the condition of a slave,
and became as men are:
and being as men are,
he was humbler yet,
even to accepting death,
death on a cross.
But God raised him high
and gave him the name
which is above all other names.
(Phil. 2:5-9)

Chapter 5
Suffering Another's Sickness

Sickness is a crisis and a challenge not only to the sick person himself, but to his loved ones as well. Facing and accepting a serious accident or disabling sickness that strikes someone who is very important to us can call for profound faith and humble courage. And the disruption that a loved one's sickness brings can call for a major revision in what we understand and expect of ourselves.

Accepting Another's Sickness

One of life's ironies is the tendency to take for granted the persons who are most important to us, especially the members of our family. Perhaps it is just as well—there is something normal and healthy about a family in which there is a certain amount of friction, and where expressions of appreciation and love are understated and not too frequent. The constant conscious awareness of how much we love and need those close to us could become maudlin and stifling.

But let a serious illness or accident strike a family member, and the others in the family become immediately and painfully conscious of how precious he is to them, of how important a role he plays in their lives. And while his sickness may affect them only indirectly, the effect it has can be profound—as much a spiritual crisis for them as it is for the sick person himself, though in a different way.

The effect is most dramatic when illness comes suddenly, or if accident strikes. We shared a leisurely cup of coffee just this morning, or we insisted that the energetic youngster wear boots to go out this snowy day. Just moments ago we spoke together, smiled and touched. And now the telephone clangs, or we hear a cry.

It is only later, after we have somehow gotten help, somehow and we can't remember how gotten to a hospital, responded automatically to questions, asked a hundred questions that all say how will he be—only later does the shock and fear that has filled our minds recede enough so we can look at it and give it a name.

Will he be all right? So alive and so present only moments ago, taken-for-granted moments, who would have thought he was so fragile? Our conscious mind reassures: of course he will be all right. It can't be terribly serious—if only because the mind cannot accept the thought that it might indeed be terribly serious. But even when the firmest and most obvious assurances have been given by doctor and hospital, our unconscious mind continues restlessly to question.

For the shock of sudden illness or accident comes not just from seeing a loved one in a moment of real danger. It comes from having to face the only too obvious but readily ignored fact that he is always vulnerable. No matter how precious he is, how important a role he plays in our lives, his strong and stready presence can be torn away in an instant, shattered like delicate crystal. The abstract, distant law that all living beings suffer and die confronts us with stark, undeniable concreteness. And the everyday surface of our lives on which we stand and walk with thoughtless confidence is suddenly shown to be woven of thin fabric indeed. A dark aloneness threatens, and we can't quite find our bearings.

In the same moment of shock that recognizes beyond words how fragile is our loved one, there is felt a nameless frustration and helplessness. We sense we are as important to him as he to us, and yet there is not one thing we can do that will really help him, or rather restore him. He enters alone into his suffering, and we are left to pace a hall, to sit restlessly in the emergency waiting room where we look up anxiously at each white-clad person who appears—always with a word for someone else. A heart attack victim is whisked from emergency to intensive care unit. The family members take turns, allowed but five minutes in an hour to be with him. It is for his own good, the conscious mind admonishes. The unconscious simmers in the anguish of helplessness. A head injury reduces a child to delirium, and even while close to him and giving first aid we cannot reach his suffering to really console him. We are helping him, doing the best we can for him, the conscious mind assures. The unconscious is choked by our utter inadequacy.

If we are the praying sort, and even if we're not, we may turn to prayer now as shock recedes and the time of our helplessness begins to move again and grow long. We may have been in the habit of kneeling every night to ask God's blessing and protection on our family members. As our easy confidence in the surface of our lives dissolves in a sort of vertigo, our easy confidence in God's protection may turn bitter for a moment. How could God allow this to happen? Doesn't God care? Is he cruel? Is he really there?

We may feel betrayed and raise angry questions to God, and then we feel guilty for asking such questions. But they are natural questions. They are again the question of Job. And out of the storm of a loved-one's illness it is possible to hear God's reply:

> Who is this obscuring my designs
>   with his empty-headed words?
> Where were you when I laid the earth's foundations?
>
> Whose command set down the laws of the heavens
>   and plotted the course of the stars?

God is there, caring and provident according to his own design and his own wisdom. There may be a bitter taste in this reminder that God is not simply the guarantee for our own expectations of health and happiness. But if as we beg God over and over again to care for our loved one, we pause just a moment to listen, we may make a discovery. God's answer is *yes.* He cares. He is caring now, and our loved one is always in his trustworthy hands.

It is a bit surprising simply to recognize that, obvious as it is in theory to one who professes to believe. And we might recognize with equal simplicity that we too are in God's hands. The irony is that God's care is there without question—our frantic questions arise from our own need to sense his presence and to trust him, rather than trusting the thin fabric on which we too heedlessly construct a taken-for-granted world, rather than judging what happens to us by the too-human measure of the surface of things.

If the intensity of our concern for our loved one does happen to bring us to prayer, and if we do respond to the crisis with trust, we may make a further discovery. Trust in God's care enables a person to relax into God's hands, and gives him a sense of being one with God, at one with the only power capable of reaching through distance or delirium, the only power capable of making some good out of our own helplessness and inadequacy. We may be able to sense that in God we are present with our loved one precisely in his suffering. Relaxing in trust then would not at all mean forgetting him. Rather our concern turns from a frantic but useless worry to a caring in which we can find strength, and in which we trust there is some real benefit for the one we're concerned about. Prayer then can override our own need for reassurance and in a real way be *for* our loved one.

Changes

The immediate crisis that is a sort of total alarm soon settles into a definite form—a specific injury, a disease with a specific name and particular characteristics. The overwhelming total shock and the radical fear it contains recedes, making way for specific challenges.

An accident, especially a burn, carries a second fear once the fear for a loved one's life is settled. A woman came to visit her husband as he recovered from burns on face and hands. At first she would enter the room and look out the window all the while they spoke. In time she could bring herself to glance at him, but it took all her courage to let her eyes rest on his scarred face. He was no longer the same as she knew him. It was a long time, even despite the wonders of plastic surgery, before she could look at him without a pang.

A disabling disease can pose an even more serious challenge. A man in his early fifties suffered a serious stroke. It left him without the use of his right side, and confined him to a wheelchair. His wife visited him regularly during his hospital stay without manifesting any serious reaction to his condition. But when the time came for him to return home, she sought a postponement, and finally admitted she couldn't face his relatively helpless condition. The hospital setting had disguised it, but she knew at home it would be painfully evident. She needed a little time and an extended period of counseling to help her accept him as he now was.

The conscious mind counsels that physical features are only on the surface, and the person remains the same however changed his appearance might be or whatever limits may now confine his activity. Armed with this conscious belief, a person may be able to suppress the feelings that naturally arise in response to the disfiguring or disabling of a loved one, telling herself that in spite of appearances he is still the same, he hasn't really changed, he hasn't really changed at all—until the conscious mind can actually ignore the change. So armed, a person can make a credible show of acceptance.

However, even though such an attitude may well enable a person to live with a loved one's disfigurement or disability, it is not really quite an acceptance but a form of denial.

For he *has* changed.

However deep and spiritual a love may be, it is always expressed in the tender gesture of a hand, a gentle smile or a glowing eye. A person is recognized as the person he is by the characteristic style for his walk, the exact way he holds his head as he stands, by the particular way he plays with his hands as he sits and talks. The deepest relationships still need the surface: that is part of being human. And so a change in the surface is a real change, and is quite naturally a cause for sorrow and for a sense of loss.

The challenge a person faces is not to see the changeless beneath the change. It is to accept the change as a real part of the person loved.

It is fairy tales that leave those who love living happily ever after in a changeless paradise. And it is romantic and sentimental movies that close with hero and heroine drifting into a brilliant sunset. Real love has an aspect called fidelity, an aspect that on reflection presents a rather frightening challenge to romantic love. Fidelity is a commitment to love another person as he is—and since he is a living, growing, changing being, as he will become. To pledge love is therefore to cast oneself into an unknown future, a future that can't be predicted or controlled without suppressing the freedom of the person loved. Fidelity means loving a changing person. Perhaps that is the significance of the traditional formula of the marriage vows, "for richer, for poorer, in sickness and in health." But it is as well an aspect of every faithful human relationship.

Fidelity in any relationship means a readiness to accept a person no matter how he changes. But how can a person pledge such a thing? How can he count on his ability to adapt and to accept anything that may happen? Sometimes such a pledge is made without trepidation, naively, and only later does the cost of fidelity become apparent. But a pledge of fidelity that is conscious of its meaning would almost have to be grounded in an act of faith. I know I reach beyond my grasp, but I trust the loving kindness of God to measure challenges to my powers, or if the challenge is greater to strengthen me accordingly. I know that the one I love is free to change and change seriously, but I trust him to God's guidance, and read God's call in whatever comes. Those who love can discover that they are together in God's hands in any crisis, rooted in that stable ground that is too deep for any change to disturb. Fidelity is a real possibility because God is faithful.

Sorrow and a sense of loss at the change accident or illness brings is very real. But at the same time it is possible to find through it a sense of renewal, and disappointment can be balanced by an unexpected, deeper fulfillment. There is a certain joy in recognizing and accepting a painful reality, for in the acceptance one can touch in a concrete way the sustaining presence of God.

Prolonged illness

The shock that marks a serious accident or sudden illness is muted when a person has an illness whose symptoms are not immediately obvious. Perhaps all he notices is a certain tiredness, a loss of weight or appetite. Perhaps he feels perfectly fit, but a routine medical examination reveals the beginnings of serious illness.

There is shock at such a diagnosis, to be sure. But the shock of sudden illness responds to its undeniable reality, while here the shock is tinged with incredulity. There must be some mistake. Or the illness is accepted as an abstraction, and life goes on as before—at least until more obvious symptoms begin to appear.

The call to acceptance is less immediately demanding than with sudden illness. There the full reality of the illness presents itself at once, and once met the challenge is overcome. But just as it is easier to dive headlong into a cold spring-fed lake than to wade in inch by shivering inch, so there is a mercy in sudden illness that is not there to aid the acceptance of a prolonged, gradual illness. The diagnosis is the first challenge, but that is abstract. Then the undeniable signs appear. Then a person watches helplessly as a loved one gradually deteriorates. The pain of loss is multiplied, and the courage to accept needs constant deepening and renewal.

A life-threatening disease like cancer may be caught in time to arrest or even cure it. And so life can return to normal, though some disfigurement may have resulted from the disease. But a quiet anxiety remains: what if the disease should recur? Just beneath the surface of consciousness there simmers the clear awareness of a loved one's vulnerability. It becomes impossible to relax again on the taken-for-granted surface of life, and the unspoken anxiety may begin to manifest itself in depression, in a growing irritability or restlessness, or even in illness. Recognizing concretely and accepting the vulnerability of a loved one is not easy.

Here, without the dramatic anguish of sudden illness that can bring a person almost in spite of himself to prayer, the way to the recognition of God's presence may be slower and more subtle. There is time now to question more seriously, time to grow angry with a God who is called omnipotent but from all appearances stands idly by, indifferent to a loved one's deterioration or danger. And God's response has no sudden storms from which to be heard, but can only be recognized as a quiet presence that remains steadfast while a person wrestles with his own inner thoughts. There is no hierophany, no flash of light. But there may come the almost embarrassed realization that the God a person has begged, questioned, scolded and cried for has been there in silent care all along.

The unconscious

A very promising young man of seventeen was driving on an errand for his parents when his car was hit head on. He suffered severe head injuries, and though his vital functions continued without complication he remained paralyzed and unconscious. Further hospitalization appeared to offer no benefit, since the care he needed could be provided at home. And so his family received him home again, caring for a still and silent son and brother over a period of ten years, until death finally came. There was no question of extremely expensive medication or life-support machinery. It was simply a matter of caring and waiting.

The special challenge faced by this family was expressed clearly enough by a question that came up only too naturally: why do you bother?

The serious ethical issue of euthanasia lurks beneath that

question. But since the boy's vital functions continued without artificial support and he required only routine care, the thought of leaving him to die never entered the family's minds. It was never a question of not bothering to care. But the question of *why* remained: what good is there in caring for him? What meaning could it have? Or is it just a prolonged absurdity?

One factor that motivated the family was hope. The medical prognosis could not absolutely exclude the possibility that he might someday return to consciousness or regain some ability to function on a higher level. But the medical basis of their hope was exceedingly slight. The possibility of a miraculous healing remained in the back of their minds, though they ceased praying directly for that after a relatively short time.

Another factor was a profound fidelity to their son and brother. He was there, and their love for him as he had been, and now as he really was, remained strong. For as long as he lived, he was a genuine presence to them despite his stillness. The members of the family developed a sense of the depth and mystery of the human person. Though he manifested no awareness, they felt it was quite possible that some kind of spiritual process was going on within him, and that some kind of communication with him was occurring. So they spoke to him as they cared for him, and sometimes just came into his room for a visit.

And they were sustained by a strong, simple faith. They believed God had his purpose in whatever happened, and so he must have some purpose in this. Sensing again that some spiritual process might well be going on deep within him, they prayed for him, and felt their care was worthwhile, since that mysterious process their care allowed could be of everlasting significance for their son and brother. As time went on, they recognized in themselves qualities and depths developing as a result of their care for him, and saw God's hand at work in their own inner lives through their situation.

That is not to say that their acceptance came without struggle, or that each member of this family did not have to wrestle with the natural question, why? What is the good? But each learned to entrust himself to God's hands, and each let go of the habit of judging what happens according to the too human measure of the surface of things.

Death

Unspoken within the acceptance of a loved one's vulnerability, disfigurement, or deterioration is the recognition of his mortality—that at any moment a person who is vitally important to us, on whom we depend in a hundred ways, may simply be gone, to all appearances disappearing into utter nothingness. The time comes though when the unspeakable becomes fact and a loved one's death is an undeniable reality.

The rituals of mourning occupy the empty hours that follow a loved one's death. Funeral directors soothe as they guide one's choice of casket, flowers and limousine. Friends and relatives gather to salute the departed and support the bereaved with their sympathetic presence. Prayers are said. Slightly unbelievable praise for the deceased is heard. Words of consolation are spoken that have been spoken countless times before. Blankets of artificial grass conceal the simple frankness of the dirt at graveside. There comes an awkward ending, and we return home, alone.

The conscious mind has a thousand consolations. He is in heaven now. God has taken him home. He's singing with the angels. His troubles are over. But as one enters a familiar room without the familiar presence, these conscious consolations fall flat and have the metallic taste of canned goods. The unconscious knows only that he is gone.

A too-easy confidence in immortality, consoling as it may be to the conscious mind, can lure a person into a denial of the reality of death that bears little resemblance to the Christian hope for resurrection. It is the anguish of death that leads to the joy of resurrection. Without that there is only an abstract hope in a bland immortality, or else an illusory conviction that the loved one never really died at all.

Probing that anguish may lead us to insight.

A genuine love for another person is never a temporary thing. The intertwining of lives penetrates the spirit of those who love, building a sense of one another's indestructible value that is deeper than any abstract conviction. Otherwise a relationship would never grow deeper than convenience and mutual entertainment, for no one dares to entrust his very self to a fragile vessel. Such a love is grounded beneath consciousness in a kind of hope: no mere physical accident like death can reach this *being*, no mere force of time can touch this absolutely precious *value*. To love, says the philosopher Gabriel Marcel, is to say you, you in particular, will never die.

But such a love simply contradicts the facts. He died. He is gone. Everything he did and everything he was exists now only in memory.

True. Love is no stranger to realism. It sees through the mortician's expert cosmetics and feels the coldness of the flesh beneath. It senses the dirt beneath the artificial grass. And it knows and feels acutely and without question that the loved one is gone, beyond our power to call him back. Love faces the facts, and so genuine love suffers anguish.

It is in the face of the facts, into the teeth of our knowledge of the facts and of our anguish at real loss, that hope affirms itself. For such hope is not founded in fact. It is grounded in the creative power of God, which is not bound by human reality and is no slave to facts. This is the power that brought light and life forth out of nothingness in the beginning, and that manifested itself in the resurrection of Christ. Hope does not touch this ground easily, for to take grace for granted is to miss it completely. It reaches that depth through the anguish of human loss and human helplessness. Christian hope does not speak of an assured continuance of life, it speaks of resurrection and regeneration as a promise and a grace, a recreative gift of God. Through anguish one can encounter this grace, and so affirm with absolute confidence that death has not spoken the last word. To love is to say that even now you, you in particular, will never die.

It is possible for Christian hope to give rise on occasion to a sense of the presence of the person who has died, a mysterious kind of communication. But this sense of presence has particular characteristics. It would not lead a person to think the deceased is still a genial companion, like the woman who maintained for several years after her husband's death everyday chit-chat with him of the sort they had habitually enjoyed. It certainly bears no resemblance to the capricious and sometimes sinister ghosts of spiritualism. Rather it is a presence sensed as a gift, and a presence not of the deceased as a sort of wandering independent spirit, but as a presence within the presence of God. A sort of communion is then possible, for both the living and the dead are together in God's hands. It is possible, in other words, on occasion to sense such a presence precisely in prayer.

In any case, the anguish of loss can find consolation when it leads a person to recognize that the value and being of the loved one is held by the power of God, and the unconditional fidelity that bound them to one another rooted them, in a way perhaps beneath consciousness before but now driven to consciousness, in that same infinitely powerful ground.

That is not by any means to say that Christian hope counsels a person to cling to a lost loved one and deny the gentle healing of time and the call to return one's attention to the business of living, indeed to new relationships. Such a clinging in a sense denies that the loved one is gone, and misses the significant realization that his life is elsewhere now. Love does not simply continue—it too is transformed and becomes a quiet recollection often beneath consciousness.

The anguish of loss then can become a genuine consolation if it leads a person to a confident hope in God's promise, a trust that the loved one is held by the power of God. That power grounds not only him but our own being, so that our fidelity can be rooted in a sense of presence together in God's faithfulness.

Adjusting

Accepting a loved one's sickness in itself can be a real challenge to a person and to a family. But adjusting to the specific demands that sickness in the family bring can be equally challenging. Habits, routines, and expectations need to be adapted to cope as well as possible with the needs of the sick or to the disruption his sickness means. Hospital and medical care bring their own burden, emotional as well as financial. And very often adults who face a real challenge in bringing themselves to accept and cope with illness in the family have the added challenge of aiding children to understand, accept, and adapt to the situation.

A new normal

Unquestionably sickness brings a disruption of a hundred taken-for-granted habits, routines, and services family members perform for one another. Especially if a parent is striken, the family discovers in just how many ways they depend on that person. And if the sick person is to be cared for at home, each member of the family discovers that new demands are placed on him.

Sometimes a kind of altruism pulls a family together to cope with the immediate crisis of sickness. Friends offer help. Children show a precocious sense of responsibility. Everyone is on his best behavior—for a while. And such a response serves well to meet the demand of a sudden, short illness: the abnormal situation calls forth extraordinary powers. But when the abnormal becomes protracted, those powers soon become exhausted, and the need to return to normal is strongly felt.

But often there shall be no more normal—at least not as it was before sickness entered the family life. The adjustment called for is not merely an emergency response, but a whole new way of life.

It is especially at this point that sickness causes stress within a family. Its constant challenge can make or break the family. A generalization often made is that sickness strengthens and binds a family relationship that is already strong, but a weak relationship is strained and even destroyed by it. Such a generalization is a great help to adjustment, of course, especially since "strong" and "weak" relationships may well be defined according to their capacity to withstand the strain of sickness—which tells us a lot indeed!

But there is a significant insight contained there, especially if we consider in connection with it just what it is in a family that provides their sense of the "normal." Is it the things the family habitually do together, their routine? Supper always at 5:30. Children clear the table, Mom washes dishes, Dad works on the evening paper. Each evening has its favorite TV shows. Homework and early to bed for children before school days. Set chores, habitual activities come Saturday. Dutifully to church Sunday. Here the routine may provide a sense of stability and reliable order in a family's life. But unless there is more to their "normal" than that, the slightest disruption could set all adrift.

Is "normal" the life-style or the living conditions the family are accustomed to? A certain taken-for-granted level of convenience in the home. A habitual etiquette. An unquestioned assumption of a certain quality of food and clothing. Here a person finds himself at home in a style of environment, and the "normal" seems a little more flexible. But economic hardship and the sudden loss of services provided by a family member can stretch this situation out of shape.

Or is "normal" the love and acceptance that marks the relationship among members of the family? Here a person is at home anywhere as long as that relationship is there. And the disruption brought by sickness is likely to be felt less in terms of changed routines or conditions, but in a new way of relating within the family because of one member's special need. The family is flexible, for "normal" will be less what is customary than what the family *makes* normal. New routines are developed to serve new needs, and family members adjust their expectations to meet new conditions.

Quite naturally, though, the disruption of a habitual life style will provoke for a time a certain amount of frustration, and that in turn may cause friction among family members. The temptation may be to suppress any discontent in the name of the family's high calling to serve the sick member. We shall do our God-given duty, and do it without complaint, mind you. Or perhaps it is that we dearly love our poor sick member, and we shall sacrifice ourselves totally to serve his every need. These are noble intentions, to be sure. But they can disguise some unconscious attitudes that are less noble, and can undermine a family's capacity realistically to adjust to the demands made on them.

When a person acts out of a conscious sense of duty or of self-sacrificing love, he may on reflection discover a sinister unconscious twist in himself—a less than pleasant concern for his own self-image, now somewhat inflated. And he may discover that his actions, consciously intended to serve the sick, are occasionally inappropriate. The sick person is to rest, yes. But the oversolicitous family forbid him to get out of bed and deny him any visitors. The dutiful family meticulously maintain their patient's regimen, but fail to notice that he would really enjoy a little simple companionship. The self-sacrificing family wait on the sick person hand and foot, and fail to take his hints that he really wouldn't mind taking just a bit of responsibility for his own care. In each case the attempt to act out a noble ideal gets in the way of really responding to the sick person himself.

At the same time the very feelings of discontent smolder unexpressed. The dutiful become more rigidly dutiful, the self-sacrificing more and more conscious of sacrifice. But the open give-and-take that characterizes a healthy family relationship is endangered, because those feelings are not honestly admitted, frankly discussed, and integrated into the new normal pattern of life. Sickness presents a real challenge to a family and few challenges can adequately be met by good intentions. Mutual support based on frank, open and accepting communication at least has an even chance.

The effort to adjust to a new normal, however, has another kind of difficulty to overcome. No matter how well a family may adapt itself to a new routine or to changed conditions, they know only too well that they are no longer quite like every other family. Especially if a parent is disabled, or a prolonged illness brings the family to face an indefinite period of hardship, the family members can hardly fail to realize that many everyday conveniences, pleasures, and ambitions are simply beyond their capabilities. Dreams and projects family members once counted on evaporate. Why us? the question stirs. The family may feel a resentment toward the sick member for depriving them of what their neighbors take for granted.

There shall be no illusions of an earthly paradise for a family with a seriously ill member. Their new normal has to extend to include their expectations and their sense of what is worhwhile in life generally. And so the new normal needs a foundation that reaches deeper than the surface of things. The challenge to adjust, like the call to accept, becomes at its core a call to faith.

Guilt

It may be the case, however, that a family simply cannot manage to care for a sick member at home, even though home care might theoretically be possible.

It would be much easier if such a situation was obvious and clear. But in many cases, especially when the member concerned is older and could be served by a convalescent home, absolutely convincing cause to do so simply is not there. It is a matter of judgment, a matter of weighing the needs of the sick and the family's capacity to adjust itself, and making a decision. And whatever decision is made, the decider knows that it could as well be otherwise.

A clearly necessary hospitalization is something that *happens* to a person. A decision to hospitalize is something that one person does to or for another. And the sick person may interpret such a decision as a rejection. More likely, the decider may fear it as a rejection, as betraying or abandoning the sick. He feels guilt. And he will feel guilt whichever way he decides—guilty for abandoning the sick on the one hand, or on the other guilty for imposing hardships and stress on his family that may be beyond their capability.

Guilt is a complex feeling. It may stem from doing wrong, and so be a gnawing call to return to the right path. But it may also stem from doing less than the ideal. Of course a person would like always to do the "right thing"—then he can maintain the feeling that he is good, upright, and respectable. Such a desire to do the "right thing" could lead in this case to a dutiful or self-sacrificing attempt to undertake something that is really beyond one's capabilities. It is a painful thing to trim one's ego ideal to fit his true hat size, and recognize that he is not, after all, a paragon of virtue but a limited human being like the rest of men. That pain is a feeling of guilt in a way, but it is a call to find one's good, uprightness, and respectability in a deeper ground than his own virtue. Despite the feeling of guilt, there is a healthy realism in the ability to make a painful decision without being trapped into playing at doing the "right thing."

Hospital worries

If a sick family member is cared for in a hospital, the family does not have quite the immediate burden of adjusting to meet his needs. Different and more subtle adjustments, though, are called for. The absence of the sick person is clearly felt, all the more acutely if it is one of the parents. Concern for him becomes a heavy burden. Were he at home, concern could take tangible form in care and service, and family members could directly help him. But when he is in the hospital, concern turns inward and the family, especially the spouse, feels growing frustration because there is nothing of real significance that they can do. Visits to the hospital set the pace for a new routine. There is the travel back and forth, back and forth. Then in the hospital there is the alien feeling, sometimes reinforced by bustling hospital staff members. We are only visitors—we have no place here. There are a few minutes of inconsequential conversation, or perhaps long awkward hours filled with obvious pastimes. The feeling of uselessness is reinforced, so that a family member returns from a visit fatigued and vaguely frustrated. Visiting itself becomes a burden, and may even become a matter of sheer duty. The emotional strength of the family is sapped.

It would make a real difference to the family if they could see some tangible significance in their visit, if their concern would take a form that played a genuinely useful role in the care of the loved one. Effort and fatigue would then have an overtone of satisfaction rather than frustration, and the emotional strength of the family would be fed rather than sapped by their new routine.

Provisions can be made, depending on hospital policy, for family members to cooperate with the hospital staff in the care of a patient. At best, they can feel that they are part of a team serving him. At least they can be informed of the plan of his care, the needs he has and the method of treating his sickness. Simply the information can allow them to feel a bit more a part of what is going on, may overcome their alien feeling, and indeed reinforce their trust and respect for the hospital staff. There are some services family members may be able to perform, like bathing the sick person, taking him for a walk, or helping him to exercise. One simple but significant thing would be to eat together—the meal, especially the evening meal, is often a kind of symbol of the unity and love of the family. But even if such participation in the care of the sick is possible, the sense of relative uselessness will remain to an extent, and remains a burden the family must bear.

Money

Another gnawing worry is the financial burden of sickness. The thought of the cost of medical care is enough to cause a good deal of anxiety. If it is the breadwinner who is sick, the family has to fear a loss of income. And the hidden, taken-for-granted services performed for the family by a parent who may now be sick would add up to a considerable sum to replace. Medical insurance may well alleviate the burden of the cost of care. Disability insurance, sickness benefits or social security may compensate at least to an extent for the loss of income. But even a limited financial burden can be a cause for anxiety, and there is danger that such anxiety can paralyze the family's ability to adapt.

The financial burden of sickness can make a family feel very much alone, and very inadequate in their loneliness. The high value given to independence in our culture—even the independence of the small nuclear family from the larger circle of relatives—here shows one of its negative aspects. Each isolated family has the expectation of an independent financial security, and there is a certain reluctance to seek help from outside. The challenge of sickness here calls for a new, less fiercely autonomous sense of security, and for a kind of humility.

Fear for the future can indeed paralyze—we just don't know how we'll manage! And the detailed, patient effort to manage—which is a matter of solving one small problem at a time—is swamped by an overwhelming anxiety for the family's *entire* future. In order to be set free to deal with the details of adjustment, the members of the family need a sense of confidence in the future—a future that is not quite under control, that is out of our hands. Again the call to faith in God's care is heard, the call to entrust the future to him. And such faith can provide a sense of security quite different from that offered by the ads of insurance companies. This security can mean letting go of one's expectations, letting go of the desire for a guaranteed earthly paradise. But it is unconditional.

Asking for help, even for advice, can symbolize for a family a loss of dignity. And the old saying reinforces that it is more blessed to give than to receive. But there is a side to such a sense of dignity that is not quite pleasant, and in its extreme form may be coupled with a kind of belligerence. "We prefer to go it alone" or "We can handle it" contains a disturbing echo of the pharisee who stood so self-assured before God with his paying of tithes and his fasting. On the other hand, the ability graciously to receive a gift, to receive without the awkwardness that stems from an unconscious need to be "even," is a beautiful characteristic. It suggests a dignity rooted not in self-sufficiency but in grace, and so grateful *receiving* can be called a highly Christian gesture.

Children

Even very young children can sense when something is wrong within the family, and all children need help to understand and cope with the emotional pressures and the adjustment that they face.

Sometimes an alert and sensitive parent can ease the burden a child bears. When a man was hospitalized for a relatively minor illness, his eight-year old son began to show signs of regression, to be irritable and aggressive, and to lose his appetite. Abstract assurances that Daddy was all right did no good. Then the mother realized that the boy's older uncle, to whom he had been quite close, had been taken to the same hospital a year before to die of a heart attack. The hospital meant death to the boy. A simple telephone call to Daddy in the hospital provided a concrete reassurance to the boy, and his disturbing behavior disappeared. The effort of a parent to sense how the child interprets the situation can pay off.

Children sometimes seem to live always in the land of Oz, with a rosy view of life and a rather limited ability to cope with hardship. Parents may therefore feel it is best to shield them as much as possible from the impact of sickness. But there is a surprising resilience in a child, especially when he is secure in the love and acceptance that provides the normal condition of the home. A child can respond to the challenge to make the best of a difficult situation, and may demonstrate a responsibility and even a faith that can be an inspiration to the rest of the family.

It is important to provide opportunities and subtle encouragement for a child to express his thoughts and feelings in response to sickness, especially when sickness includes the danger of death. A young child may quietly harbor a terrifying sense of having *caused* the sickness by some misbehavior or angry thought. An older child may be torn in his effort to revise his expectations from life. Accepting and adjusting to illness is a difficult enough challenge for a mature adult. It may be overwhelming for a child. And a family that accepts and adjusts together, in a shared response to the situation, has a better chance to be strengthened by the challenge rather than torn apart by it.

Sickness, then, brings its challenges not only to the one who suffers the disease or accident, but to all who bear the burden of his illness. But sickness also brings to them its call and its promise of significance. When sickness has passed, or when the family has so adjusted that their situation is experienced fully as normal for them, they may be able to look back over their trial and recognize that they have been visited by grace.

Part III

Caring

Those who care for the sick, family members or medical professionals, are primarily persons. Caring presents emotional demands on them in addition to professional or medical responsibilities. The simplest but most challenging demand is love. Close to that is the obvious but easily overlooked fact that every patient, family member, and medical professional is a person who needs to be respected and accepted for what he is. Finally, within the caring relationship difficult ethical problems can arise that call those who care for the sick to a high degree of personal responsibility.

Chapter 6

Serving The Sick

The family with a sick member at home has a double call addressed to them. One is that difficult inner challenge to meet sickness with an attitude of positive acceptance and to adjust to its impact on each member of the family and on family life as a whole. The second is simply the call to serve the sick person.

Caring for the medical needs of the sick person is only one aspect of this call, though by no means an insignificant one. The effort to meet these needs at home links the family not only to medical professionals, but to a whole network of agencies and organizations.

Caring for the sick person as a person, though, is an ongoing responsibility no agencies, organizations, or professionals can directly share. Here the family is likely to be best qualified to serve, for what the sick person needs as a person is basically love. But that love, intense and genuine as it may be within a family, needs to be guided in order to serve the sick effectively. It needs to be guided particularly by a sensitivity to the inner needs of the sick person. The inner challenge and struggle with which sickness confronts the one who suffers it is quite often hidden or disguised. And the ability to understand and respond to his real needs is not one which every family can take for granted.

Even more sensitivity is needed in caring for the inner needs of a child, whose inner world is sometimes quite different from an adult's, and whose capacity to express himself is not fully developed. So the call to care for the sick can present a complex challenge to a family—but a challenge to grow and deepen as persons.

Meeting Medical Needs

Part of the pain of struggling to accept sickness in a loved one is the sense of helplessness and of being utterly alone. One consolation of the effort to care for the sick is that one is by no means alone, and in most cases there are a number of directions to turn for help.

Families usually turn first to medical professionals and to hospitals. Hospitals, though, are generally geared to care for the critically or acutely ill. Once the crisis is over, ongoing or routine care becomes more and more the responsibility of the family.

The transition from hospital care to home care is generally supervised by the doctor, and guidance is readily available through the doctor or through the hospital's counseling agency, enabling the family to find the help they need in serving the sick.

The family is likely to be surprised at the range and variety of agencies and organizations to which they can turn, most often without cost. Professional medical assistance is available in nearly all communities through the Visiting Nurse Association. A number of volunteer groups provide a range of assistance, from organizations that can provide specific advice and help for a particular disease to church groups whose members make themselves available to help with numberless incidental needs, even—or especially—the need for family members to be free for a few hours of shared recreation away from the burdens of sickness. The generosity and dedication of people in these groups is often truly inspiring, and provide for the family the consolation of knowing there are people to whom they can turn for help— sometimes regardless of time.

Sometimes a simple conversation can be of great help. The

family whose father faces heart surgery may be burdened with a thousand numberless fears. But volunteer organizations like the Mended Heart Club can bring this family together with people who have gone through the very challenge they face, who can advise them and help them get their fears into perspective.

A family may find it awkward to accept such help from volunteers or from publically funded agencies. Once again our society's high valuation of independence shows its negative side. That awkwardness is natural, in a way. The freedom to receive gracefully does not come automatically. Those on the giving side—the volunteers—need to be sensitive to the need of some families to repay them somehow. While money or large gifts would of course be out of the question, the volunteer also needs the ability to receive gracefully. One family presented to the woman who had helped them some delicious ethnic pastries. An Appalachian family surprised their helper with a cane they had carved with meticulous care and artistry. These gestures of thanks were filled with a simple but beautiful dignity, and they erased from the situation any awkwardness.

Serving Inner Needs

As a person, the basic need of the sick is simply love. But love is not a simple thing. Sometimes in spite of the best intentions and the deepest feelings, people can fail to communicate love. And even when a family conveys its love to its sick member, they can fail to recognize and respond to his particular inner needs.

"All you need is love"

One of the sufferings connected especially with prolonged sickness is a kind of isolation, the sense of living in a different world, a world removed from the lives and concerns of family and friends. This is the pain so subtly reinforced by the get-well card, the pain quietly manifest is a certain lack of enthusiasm or spontaneity in conversations with family and friends. To an extent some isolation is to be expected, for the sick person's world is different from the busy scheduled lives most Americans consider normal. But the pain and the intensity of loneliness connected with it can vary a great deal from one sick person to another. In a hospital, one person may have relatively few visitors, yet feel loneliness less acutely than a person with a constant stream of friends and relatives. A sick person cared for at home may not necessarily feel this pain less than a patient in a hospital. A person whose activities are severely limited by sickness may feel less isolated than one capable of a relatively wide range of activity. Number of visitors, length of time spent with visitors, place, and kind of disease do not fully explain why the pain and the intensity of loneliness can vary.

One plausible explanation of that variance points to an intangible quality of the sick person's relationship with family and friends—or perhaps of his relationship with only one person who is close to him. A good word for that intangible quality is "availability."

A clue to the nature of "availability" might be found in the definite but intangible "sense" we get about certain types of conversations. One sense is characteristic of conversations at cocktail parties or rambling over-the-back-fence talk. One person tells about a third cousin who fractured a toe when the fringe of his moccasin got caught in an escalator. That brings to the mind of the next person the case of his nephew's brother-in-law who suffered abdominal bruises when his rope bathrobe sash caught in the handrailing as he was running down stairs. And on the round goes, each person telling his story in turn, while the others listen with half their minds, but eagerly rehearse with the other half the story they eagerly wait to tell. Such a conversation is enjoyable and even entertaining. It passes the time with bits of news or interesting anecdotes. But it has the character of a series of monologues connected only by association, if at all. There is little real communication, little real listening and responding to what another person is saying. And so when the time has passed and the entertaining escape is over, the pain of loneliness can return full force. A pleasant time has been spent in company, but there has been no real sharing of persons.

Another type of conversation tries to reach deeper. Sick persons and their families may be especially familiar with it. In a hospital emergency room a family waits anxiously while a loved one receives care. The hospital chaplain stops to talk briefly with them, and he may speak words of consolation that have a well-worn and familiar sound. Family members know they are supposed to feel consoled and grateful, so they respond in those terms. But somehow the feelings seemed forced, and the end of the conversation brings less a sense of consolation than a vague feeling of relief. This kind of conversation attempts to bring about a sharing of persons, but the sharing may have a tendency to go in only one direction. Words are spoken, but the family does not feel that they have really been able to express what is within them and be understood.

But in another type conversation there may be quite a different sense. I may be talking about anything, about nothing in particular. But I sense that the person to whom I speak is really listening to me. Not only does he understand my words, but he perceives my mood and my feelings and responds to them. I feel I am welcome, that the person with whom I speak opens himself to me, gives me a place within him so that I feel at home with him. I sense gratefully that he considers me important and enjoyable in myself. He gives me his full attention. When we speak he is totally *present* to me, and his mind is not wandering or preoccupied with other affairs as we converse. Perhaps no profound sentiments are exchanged, no intimate secrets revealed, no pledges given. But I sense unquestionably that as we speak he is full *there* for me, in a sense at my disposal. I sense I can call upon him in any situation and he will respond *to me*—with enjoyment, consolation, help, advice or simply play, depending on my need. This person manifests that intangible quality of availability.

The beautiful thing about such a person is that by his openness, sensitivity and kindness he creates in himself a place where I can be at home, where I am no longer alien, a stranger. Availability by its very nature overcomes isolation, for I know I am not alone as long as this person cares for me. And that assurance is strong, remaining alive despite time and distance. Though years may pass between the occasions when we meet, each meeting begins as if only hours intervened.

It is no wonder, then, if such a quality in a relationship makes a significant difference in the degree to which a sick person suffers loneliness.

How then would someone go about developing this quality in himself?

Ironically, the selfconscious effort to develop availability defeats itself for by such effort one's attention focuses on *himself* as he relates to others, rather than focusing on the other. But an awareness of its characteristics may help a person to grow toward it, or at least recognize in himself the need to grow.

Availability is marked for one thing by an ability to give one's full attention to another person. That is not as simple as it sounds. For most people have, quite normally, a tendency toward a subtle division in attention. We attend directly to the other person, but indirectly we are aware of ourselves. We tend to see the other in terms of how he touches our world rather than stepping out of our own world to understand and appreciate him as he is in himself. Our awareness of him therefore tends to be selective, as if we pass the other through a filter and admit into our mind only part of him, the part that relates to our concerns. We hear and respond to the words he speaks, but unless we can understand a bit the world of experience and the point of view out of which he speaks, we will not be able to hear what is unsaid, to respond to the intention or the feeling beneath the words. Availability means the capacity to let go for a moment of one's self and one's own perspective, to yield oneself to the other person and be at his disposal. So availability calls for a readiness to let go that has spiritual roots near the readiness to accept suffering and even to face death: the capacity to empty oneself.

Availability is also marked by the ability to share one's own world with another person. A person may open his world and his heart to the best of listeners, but unless the listener in turn shares his world and heart, that person has the uncomfortable feeling of a poker player who has laid his cards on the table while the other player holds his cards close to his chest. But sharing one's own world is not such an easy thing either. Sharing surface concerns and everyday chatter is not difficult, and may serve well as a preliminary stage in a deeper relationship. But there is a certain healthy hesitancy to share thoughts and feelings that make up one's inner world. Perhaps a person naturally senses that those thoughts and feelings could easily be misunderstood or abused, and so sharing them means taking a risk—or rather calls for trust in the other person. To share one's feelings is in a way to place oneself—if only a little—in the hands of the other person. It is a high compliment really. The risk is intensified and the compliment is amplified if the thoughts and feelings happen to be unpleasant, or imply a criticism of or demand on the other person. But a sensitive frankness too is part of availability, and the ability to be open about less pleasant things is something of an indicator of the real honesty of a relationship.

Availability then is a quality in a relationship that makes it creative. It makes possible a sharing of persons, and so can overcome isolation and loneliness. It is sensitive and sympathetic, but frank and objective. By such availability, a person very clearly but indirectly communicates love, and he is well on the way toward recognizing and responding to the particular inner needs of the sick person for whom he cares.

Some particulars

If the basic inner need of the sick person is simply love, it is a need he shares with every other human being. But his situation—sickness, disability, pain and like—give a particular shape to that need. He needs acceptance and reassurance about his situation, he needs a patient and sympathetic listener for his complaints, and he needs to be able to participate significantly in the world about him.

The sick person, as we have seen, faces a difficult challenge in accepting and adjusting to his sickness, especially if it is prolonged, disabling, or disfiguring in any way. The home setting may actually intensify his difficulty, for the familiar surroundings bring into sharper relief any loss of his accustomed ability or mobility. Often his struggle to accept and adjust goes on without words, perhaps without a clear and direct awareness of the cause or significance of his distress. Those who care for him therefore need to be alert and sensitive to his hidden needs, and to see his situation as much as possible from his point of view.

The sick person needs acceptance and reassurance. Especially if he is disabled or disfigured, he needs to know concretely that he is accepted as he now is. Words just may not be able to do the job. A hug or a tender holding of his hand may convey love and acceptance that is deeper than words. One man who had lost a hand confessed that he felt rejected by his wife in spite of kind words because she would never look at the marks of his injury. Consolation came for him in a poignant episode when he brought her to look at and touch the injured area. Acceptance came with tears, to be sure, but then it was real.

He may need reassurance to help him calm anxieties and fears about his illness. There is nothing less reassuring, though, than a vague affirmation that "everything's going to be all right." The sick person's fears may be quite specific, and vague generalities communicate to him an evasion or a lack of concern. Real reassurance must arise from a clear understanding of what is being reassured. If a sick person is anxious about his condition, the one who speaks to him needs to know what his condition is, and communicate that to him, without evasion or denial, to the extent the sick person can understand it and cope with it. But it may happen that the sick person, especially if he is a child, has filled his mind with erroneous or even fantastic fears about what is wrong with him, perhaps from reading and misguided self-diagnosing, or perhaps from observing other sick people. The most objective reassurance concerning his actual condition is not likely to console him unless he is given the chance to express those fears and have them directly met. Reassurance can set false fears to rest. But trying to cover over well-founded anxieties is a disservice, perhaps even a betrayal of the sick person. He needs nothing less than support for a delusion; what he needs is support and strength in his struggle to accept and adjust to reality.

The sick person needs a patient and sympathetic listener for his complaints. Here the quality of availability is especially important, for if we hear the complaints without understanding the world of experience out of which they are spoken, we will tire easily of them and even find them very irritating. We need to be alert to what is *unsaid* in complaining. We need to probe the suffering or anxiety that lies beneath it.

Complaining is a normal outlet for pain and stress, and it serves as a call for help in overcoming the causes of that pain and stress. Sometimes it arises from an easily identifiable source: a bedridden person complains of a lump in the bed. Investigation reveals a sheet pulled loose at the corner and bunched up in the middle. Straightening the sheet removes the lump, and the sick person's complaint gives way to a sigh of relief. But sometimes the causes of the pain and stress are complex or are hidden deep within the struggle to cope with sickness. Stages along the path to acceptance may express themselves in complaining. Anger and frustration at being sick—indeed at the limits of the finite human condition—seek tangible targets in whatever and whoever is at hand. An unconscious fear of rejection might prompt a sick person's complaints, so that they signify his effort to test and prove his family's acceptance of him. Anxiety over the possibility of death may be the unconscious reason why the sick person may demand endless attention and infallible care. In any case, the family may find themselves beseiged by criticism, worries, and even unreasonable demands.

How shall they respond? Anger and irritation at the complainer is a normal enough response, but it is a response to the surface and fails to hear what is unsaid beneath. Obsequious efforts to meet every demand prove counterproductive, for they fail to reach the hidden cause of the complaint and they disguise a growing irritation that can erupt eventually into serious conflict. They may desperately choose to ignore the complaining—which leaves the sick person alone with his anxieties.

The sick person needs to be listened to. That means more than simply sitting there and "taking it." He needs help to reach the hidden source of his pain and stress. He needs help gradually to bring his unconscious anxieties and fears close enough to his conscious awareness that he can recognize them and come to terms with them. There is a relatively clear way family members—or at least one who is close to the sick person—can serve him in this need. We can listen to him, and then as far as possible discuss his concern with him. We can first reflect back to him our understanding of what he is saying. This gives him an opportunity to correct us if we misunderstand him. But it also allows him to take an objective look at what he is saying, recognize it and perhaps discover that this is not really his concern. By acting as a sympathetic reflector and interpreter of his own thoughts, we can help him toward a conscious understanding of anxieties or pains that are so close to him he can't see them clearly by himself. But further, we can by our own understanding of the kinds of inner stresses he may be suffering guide him gently and sensitively toward discovering the source of his pain and coping with it. In one family, the sick son insisted that a family member be always present at home. It was not an unreasonable demand, but discussing it in this way brought the young man's intense anxiety about death to the surface, and gave his parents and the doctor an opportunity to reassure him and set his fears to rest.

The sick person needs to be able to participate significantly in the world around him. He needs to be allowed to share in the world of his loved ones, and he needs to have some sense of responsibility for himself and of contributing to others.

Family members in their concern for the sick person may be tempted to shield him from any stress or unpleasantness they face. Well-intentioned as this effort may be, it tends to produce an effect opposite what the family desires. For the sick person is likely to have enough common sense to know there are stresses, however rosy and untroubled a picture he is given. And so he senses that he is being excluded from an important part of his family's life. And the sick person is likely to care very deeply about his family, so that sense of exclusion is painful and may even give rise to imagined worries much more serious than the real ones from which he is sheltered. For if he is not allowed to share whatever real burdens the family faces, what is he likely to imagine but that *he* is their burden, and one too heavy to talk about at that?

A sensitive frankness between the sick person and his family allows him to share their real world. He knows his sickness demands an adjustment on their part, so constructively sharing that effort and maybe the strain it involves reveals no great secret. Of course *complaining* to the sick person about the trouble he causes would be destructive indeed. But giving him the opportunity to share the family's concerns gives him a real place in his family no matter how disabled he might be.

The sick person also needs to be able to take some real responsibility in his family and to make a positive and tangible contribution to their life. If he is pampered, waited on hand and foot, and allowed to do nothing to take care even of his own slightest needs, he may well get the message that he is considered a vegetable, with nothing at all to contribute to his family. Especially if he formerly made a major contribution to them, he is likely to resent such treatment and even rebel at it. The sick person—particularly if he suffers from a prolonged illness or is disabled—wants to live a life as close to normal as possible. He wants to be as independent as he can be, at least in meeting his own personal needs. It may well be that the range of things he can do is severely limited. But he needs his family to respect what capacities he has and to allow him to care for himself as much as he can.

Most often there are many ways he can contribute to the ongoing life of his family, within the limits imposed by his sickness. One mother was confined to a wheelchair, but in time and with the understanding and cooperation of her family rearranged the household so that she could resume the bulk of housekeeping duties. A father was confined to bed, but from there managed the family finances, as well as helping his children with homework and whatever needs they brought to him. Further, the sick person's judgment and thinking is likely to be unimpaired, and so he may be perfectly capable of participating fully in family decisions.

But there are also many significant but unexpected contributions the sick person can make. One man confined to bed had learned leatherwork through the hospital's occupational therapy program. He enjoyed making little gifts for his family, indeed gifts made with real artistry, and he shared with them his enjoyment of his new skill. A partially paralyzed woman with two teen-aged children became an avid reader of quality novels, and her enthusiasm brought her children to become acquainted with writers like Melville and Dostoevsky. But the greatest unexpected contribution may be a much more subtle one. A laboring man after his disabling accident met the challenge to accept and adjust to his new condition, and his spiritual struggle and the depth it gave to him became a leaven in the life of his family. His children came to know a gentle sense of humor, a practical wisdom, and a depth of faith that was a treasure for them.

Yes, the sick person needs to take responsibility in the family and to make a contribution. It might appear that he himself has to make the first move, to ask to share, to reach for responsibility, to give. But he would never be able to begin if it were not for a kind of availability on the part of his family. For the sick or disabled person is not all that confi-

dent in himself and is not all that likely to assert himself
without support and encouragement. The man who did
leatherwork for his family had found the craft very boring in
the hospital, for it had no meaning or value except to pass the
time. What gave it meaning was his young daughter's delight
in a little purse he made for her. From then on his family's
genuine interest and appreciation encouraged him to develop
what turned out to be a real knack for artistry in leather. And
the man whose acceptance of his disability and his simple
spiritual depth inspired his family came to that acceptance
and depth through a struggle his family shared. They were
interested in him, genuinely eager to enter his world and bring
him into theirs. The contribution which benefits both the sick
and those about him grows out of a relationship marked by
availability on the part of both.

Caring For The Sick Child

The basic inner need of the sick child is simply love. But
again love is not a simple thing. The child needs his parent's
presence and support more the younger he is, and his parents
need to be especially sensitive to be able to see into his world.
He needs help to accept and cope with his sickness, and to
keep up a relationship with the world of others that is as
normal as possible.

A younger child—from the age when he first recognizes his
parents even to school age—depends on his parents for his
orientation, for his sense that things are all right and he will
be secure. Sickness and especially hospitalization will be
disturbing enough for him even with his parents present—but
if he is separated from them the experience may be traumatic.
Some hospitals allow and even encourage a parent to room in
with the sick child unless medical reasons forbid it, at least
until the child comes to know members of the staff. The
presence of his parents gives him strength and support in his
sickness. As a child grows older, the actual physical sense of

their availability—that intangible quality in a relationship—
can support him even in their absence.

The particular inner fears, struggles and sufferings of the
sick child may be hidden beneath apparently insignificant
questions, and within the child's play. Sensitive listening and
alert observation can reveal those fears, struggles and sufferings. A rather quiet four-year-old entered the hospital for a
tonsillectomy. She seemed to have no trouble adjusting to the
new surroundings as she awaited surgery. But in her play she
acted out the coming operation on her doll. Very businesslike,
she sliced with a toy knife across the doll's neck and said,
"There. That's it. You're dead," and threw the doll aside. That
revealed the child's intense but hidden fears to her mother,
who was able to reassure her by explaining more clearly just
what would happen to her in the operating room. A hospitalized boy of six calmly asked his father if someone would come
get him in case the hospital caught fire. The father realized
that fire may not have been the question: the boy probably
feared *death*, a destroying force that might trap him like fire.
Had he stopped at reassuring his son that a fire in the hospital
was unlikely, the boy's fear would have remained. But he sat
and talked with him, discovering his hidden fears and helping
the boy deal with them.

The kind of fears that lie just beneath the surface of the sick
child's mind may be quite different from those of an adult, for
the adult generally has some rather specific idea of his
condition and of what to expect. A child is most likely
bewildered at sudden changes in his surroundings, at being
restricted in activity, at being simply unable to do what may
have been an easy matter not long before. And that bewilder-
ment leads to anxiety: something is wrong—with me! I don't
know what it is and there's nothing I can do about it. A child
from age three to about school age may tend to feel guilty for
his condition—as if he is being punished for something he did
wrong. Except he has no idea what it is. Or he may feel guilt
for some small crime like cookie-stealing and feel hopeless
and doomed because nothing he does removes the punish-

ment and restores his normal relationship with his parents. An older child may feel hopelessly cut off from others, like some kind of freak, develop a sense of insecurity about his ability to succeed as a person, and so withdraw socially more and more. If a parent is alert to what concerns his child, if he can get inside the sick child's inner world a bit, then he may be able to provide a great deal of help in meeting those fears.

The child needs help in accepting his sickness. A big part of that may be helping to see sickness for what it is, and to overcome the fears and misunderstandings that magnify it. A clear and understandable explanation of his sickness and his treatment may be a help. But most important is listening, helping the child to express his concerns and fears, and reassuring him accordingly. There may be a temptation to hide the truth from a child, especially if he faces prolonged illness or disability. But the child will sense that something is seriously wrong and the anxiety of not knowing, of knowing something is hidden from him, will magnify his fear. A child may be quite capable of facing a hard reality and accepting it, and calling on him to make the best of a hard situation may bring forth surprising maturity and strength.

The child needs to be included in the world that surrounds him, too. He lacks the inner resources of the adult, and has not yet developed habits of using time and occupying himself, the habits that give some order the life of an adult. The sick child needs help here: some sort of order and predictability in his routine, a variety of activities to occupy him, and the response and appreciation that gives those activities significance. The school-age child especially needs to preserve his contacts with his friends, to share their schoolwork, play with them to the extent that is possible, to show them what he likes to do, and things he may have made.

But there are days when the emotional burden of illness demands its due, and the sick child may become despondent or depressed. Overly-optimistic predictions of recovery may lead to disappointment, and setbacks may cause the child to wonder if he'll *ever* recover. The orderly routine may have to be set aside for a day, and maybe a little bit of special attention is called for. But sickness remains a struggle, and parents need to be careful that the child's ability to act with purpose is not dissipated.

With such help, a child may be able to profit from his sickness. The discipline of the struggle can develop patience and a sturdy sense of being in command of one's mind and heart. The value of friendship is intensified. And the bond of genuine love with his family is strengthened.

The challenge to care for the sick can therefore call a family to reach a depth of love and an appreciation for one another that they might never have known otherwise. They may share intimately in the spiritual process that occurs within sickness, a process that thinly veils the mysterious workings of God in the life of a human person. They share in the work of God— indeed sometimes they may sense his active presence in the quiet process of healing, either physical or spiritual. Perhaps then there is a significance for the family of a sick person in an aspect of the New Testament: as Jesus proclaimed the coming of the kingdom of God to men, the way he dramatically portrayed the presence of God's realm was precisely by the spiritual and physical healing of the sick.

Chapter 7
Professionals and People

The first impression a person receives upon looking at today's health care professionals and institutions is one of incredible complexity. If he walks into a single urban hospital, he is for a while simply bewildered by the size of the place, the number of departments, and the apparent intensity and variety of activity. If he goes to study the national health care picture, he is overwhelmed by an increasing variety of specializations, an ever-developing technology, or simply the organizational complexity within hospitals, regional hospital systems, professional organizations, and centers of education and research.

It is too easy to overlook in all this complexity the simplest aspect of health care—and perhaps the most important. Within the research centers and organizations and specializations, behind the white brick walls and the glass-and-steel doors of the hospitals, people are doing their best to care for people.

It is easy to overlook the human dimension of health care. But that oversight can have unfortunate results. If medical professionals forget that their patients are people they may reinforce the sense of alienation and isolation that adds such pain to illness, and they may even hinder the process of healing that they are supposed to be helping. If patients and families forget that medical professionals are people, they may have unreasonable expectations and make unreasonable demands, and so they may even interfere with the doctors' and nurses' efforts to care for them. And if medical professionals forget that they themselves are people, they may cause subtle but serious harm to their relationships with the people they would serve.

To understand medical professionals as people, we need first to examine critically some of the sterotypes that affect the way we think of them and sometimes the image they may have of themselves. Then we should try to understand some of their burdens and some of the limits within which they work.

Recognizing that patients and their families are people should in turn affect the quality of doctors' and nurses' relationships with them. As persons, patients and families need to be given responsibily, to be kept informed, and to have their inner needs taken seriously into account.

Medical Professionals Are People

The medical profession has generally been held in very high regard within the American culture. As a profession, medicine has had a great deal of tangible success and has made dramatic progress in conquering diseases and minimizing the long-term effects of illness or accident. Indeed the medical professional, especially the doctor, is given a role as hero in our popular culture. He rivals the detective as a source of prime time television excitement. But even the detective is silent before his infallible scientific wisdom, and the television audience waits outside the glowing doors of the operating room with a reverence and sense of expectation reserved in ancient times for the high-priest's secret rites within the Holy of Holies. In a secular age skeptical of the Bible's word, advertisers find ready acceptance for any statement made by an actor wearing a white coat, or prefaced by the magisterial formula "doctors recommend." In an age for which God is a question and Science is the answer, it appears that medicine is the special incarnation of Science. New discoveries— especially breakthroughs toward curing frightening diseases—are the miracles of the modern world, generating excitement and reverence that find close parallels from the medieval world in the awe and expectation that surrounded the saint with a reputation for working wonders. And in an age in which secular salvation is a full life in an earthly paradise, the priest to whom the faithful turn for the sacraments of that salvation is the doctor.

The success of medicine is very real, and the reverence in which the profession has been held is no doubt gratifying. But it has its dark side, a poisonous aspect that medical professionals sense with increasing concern.

For one thing, living up to a reputation for miracle-working is not the easiest thing in the world to do. The patient may think the doctor is capable of infallible and virtually instantaneous cures, and the complete elimination of pain. (After all, television diseases are always healed in the half-hour or hour time slot, minus commercials of course.) And so the doctor finds himself called on to meet unrealistic and sometimes fantastic demands. And if the patient expects his doctor to have powers bordering on the supernatural, the slightest failure or hint of uncertainty on the doctor's part may shatter his patient's confidence, and even arouse anger—as if a merely competent doctor was an imposter.

A poison even more insidious may affect the doctor's image of himself. Revered like a priest, the medical professional may be tempted into a sort of clericalism, especially in his relationship to nonprofessionals. He possesses the sacred powers and the special knowledge, couched indeed in a Latin jargon. He refers to nonprofessionals as "laymen." But most seriously, he may habitually keep from a patient and family the kind of information that would enable them to exercise a genuinely responsible role in care, denying them the opportunity to make informed and significant decisions. Of course the capacity of the family to understand and to participate in patient care will be limited. But there is a faint stink of clericalism in a doctor's failure to make room for patient and family participation in care, especially if that has the practical effect of holding them in unquestioning dependence on him.

A further danger arises if medical professionals unconsciously share the assumption that salvation is a full life in an earthly paradise, or that life is the one absolute value. For where salvation is at stake, the one thing necessary is in question, there is no counting the cost.

And so it sometimes happens that highly expensive measures are taken to prolong only for a few days the life of a patient who is unquestionably about to die, and that without full consultation with the family. Or on a smaller scale, treatment that is not really necessary may be recommended or simply given without any mention to patient or family of the cost involved and without giving them an opportunity for decision.

Where such attitudes are common among doctors and health care institutions, a person may find himself placed in a very frustrating situation. In a sizeable midwestern city, a woman became anxious about recurring stomach pains. Though she and her family had lived in the city over a year, they were unable to obtain a family doctor because the general practitioners in the area refused to take new patients unless they underwent a lengthy and expensive physical examination—which this family could not then afford. Disturbed by a particularly painful episode, she went to the emergency room of their city's Catholic hospital. There she spent over two hours, and the pain subsided without treatment. She was asked questions, tests were administered without informing her of their nature and purpose, and the emergency room doctor stopped for about two minutes, spent mostly in small talk. A week later a bill arrived for well over fifty dollars, including a fee for emergency service, a separate and higher fee for the doctor, and a substantial lab fee, charges for tests some of which the woman had no idea were being made. For all this she was none the wiser, for no diagnosis was ever conveyed to her. Needless to say, she and her family felt some resentment toward the hospital and the doctor as a result of this experience.

Such medical clericalism can have a poisonous effect on the relationships between doctor and patients in at least two ways. First, the failure to inform a patient adequately and give him responsibility in decisions affecting his care can bring about a sense of alienation, of being excluded, that can undermine trust. Second, to the extent that experiences like the above become no longer exceptional, a more generalized sense of resentment could well arise—a kind of anticlerical sentiment in reaction to unnecessarily high costs which patient and family are powerless to control. The respect with which patients generally regard their doctors could turn to suspicion, seriously hampering the good work of the medical profession.

It is important then to medical professionals that their common humanity be kept in mind—by themselves as well as by their patients and prospective patients. Forgetfulness of that humanity—consoling or flattering as it may be in the short run—carries with it a long term risk of undermining the trust so essential to the medical professionals' effectiveness.

But mindfulness of that humanity carries with it a challenge of its own.

For it may well be that a patients' life itself is at stake. If he perceives his doctor as a wonder-worker endowed with infallibility, trust comes easily—but it is a fragile trust. However, if he perceives his doctor as a person—competent indeed but hardly infallible—he may be alarmed to realize that he is called on to place his very life in the hands of a mere human being. Now trust comes less easily.

How can a person consciously trust his very life to the hands of another person, especially if there is serious risk involved?

One person may take the attitude of a gambler playing the odds. Perhaps he faces an operation to remove what may be a malignant growth. He looks at his options, and each of them is risky. And so he places his bet on the surgeon. But in effect he is not trusting the surgeon with his life—that risk he leaves to chance. What he does count on is the doctor's ability to provide the best chance for him. He will therefore be concerned about the doctor's competence, almost like the bettor at the race track who checks a horse's track record. And so for him the surgeon simply has to function, the more like a predictable machine the better.

Another person, though facing a similar situation, may take an attitude that is less stoic but at the same time less impersonal. He realizes that his life may well be in the balance, and he is frankly afraid. He takes the prospect of death with full seriousness. In trusting his doctor, however, this person may come to recognize and accept the tragic fragility of the human situation, where what is incomparably precious—life itself—hangs from moment to moment upon slender threads, weak and fallible human beings providing for one another's needs. The slightest error and even the simple limits of human possibilities may mean the loss of life. There is no guarantee, no insurance to reduce the risk. But that is after all what it means to be a human being—to be finite and so always to have one's life and everything one holds dear radically beyond his control. There is no guarantee, and so such a person might be filled with terror at the thought of confronting death. But then again he may be drawn to realize that human reality has a ground where death is not absolute, that there is one in whose hands life is secure—though in a way beyond the imaginable, through and beyond the dark mystery of death. This person's trust is not the gambler's calculated odds, nor a sort of "sure bet" with guaranteed winnings of prolonged life on one hand and a taken-for-granted immortality on the other. This person's trust is grounded in a faith that God is acting in what happens, and that God's call is found in the very fragility of the human condition. Yes, this surgeon is a man. Finite himself, he too hangs upon slender threads—now, upon the steadiness of hand and eye. And this patient trusts his life to these hands— a man's hands like his own—perhaps with a sense of wonder at the profound responsibility given to fragile men in this world. This person's trust then amounts to a humble embrace of the human condition, grounded in faith that God's presence is there for him, veiled but sure, in whatever occurs. And part of that embrace is a genuine but realistic appreciation for his doctor as a human being.

The doctor to whom so many may trust their lives has reason himself for fear at such a profound responsibility. Indeed, if he were to fill his mind with how much depends on him, he might become mentally paralyzed, unable to act effectively at all. On the other hand, if he becomes deluded with an absolute confidence in his own competence, he could lose his sense of caution and self-criticism, and discover the fallibility of his common humanity too late—perhaps at the cost of needless loss of life. The doctor too needs to accept the fragility of the human condition, and to wonder at the profound responsibility that he himself has been given. His confidence then would find firm ground in the presence with him of the One who has ultimately given him that responsibility. And so as he enters the operating room to perform an operation, he enters as fully competent as it is possible for him to be, but with a confidence grounded deeper than mere human competence—an attitude perhaps like an unspoken prayer.

The nurse

When serious sickness tears a man out of the world he is used to and flings him into a hospital, that hospital becomes for a while the world in which he must live. And as that while grows longer, more and more he has to find in this new and smaller world ways to deal with his complex and varied inner needs.

Though the doctor has the primary responsibility for the patient's medical care, it is the nurse who cares for him most immediately and constantly. When the patient needs something, his call is answered by the nurse. When the patient's family visits, it is usually the nurse who talks with them about his care. And it is the nurse on whom falls the unpredictable and complex burden of helping the patient deal with his inner needs. So in addition to her role in his medical care, she may be called upon to act as counselor, confidant, lifter of drooping spirits, liaison between doctor and family, and sometimes friend. Besides competence as a medical professional, she finds demanded of her an inner resourcefulness and—what may be most difficult—a capacity for a delicate emotional balance in her complex relationships.

Nurses are people caring for people, and inevitably the nurse is drawn to place an emotional investment in her patients. Sometimes that very human concern can become an obstacle, as the nurse may tend to identify too closely with her patient, especially if the patient's age and circumstances are similar to her own. A young woman who faced serious surgery became fearful and upset as the time of her operation drew near. Her young nurse so shared her fear that she too became upset, and *both* had to be consoled by another nurse who was older and a bit wiser. In the intensive care unit of a small city's hospital, one shift of nurses began to show signs of extraordinary emotional strain. The hospital chaplain discovered that they were identifying so strongly with their critically ill and dying patients that they would go through the emotional struggle of facing, fighting, or finally accepting death with each patient. No wonder they were under a strain.

Fearful of such overinvolvement—or perhaps scarred because of it—a nurse may tend to the opposite extreme, a cold detachment that avoids any emotional investment in the patient. Disguising itself as professional objectivity, such detachment comes closer to depersonalizing the nurse-patient relationship. Since the patient is likely to have a very real need for human contact, what the nurse intends as professionalism registers with him as coldness or as positive disregard. Again the nurse's effectiveness is jeopardized.

The nurse is called upon to walk the delicate emotional balance between becoming overly involved and becoming depersonalized. This is no easy feat, especially because it is more than likely that her preparation has emphasized technical competence, perhaps without bringing her to an awareness of the mystery of her own inner self. Each nurse meets this challenge in her own way, and each deals with it uniquely. But if she is going to keep her balance, she will need to recognize and accept two aspects of the human condition that touch her closely. The first is the limited nature of her relationship with her patient. The second is the radical limit of finiteness itself.

The relationship of nurse to patient is a role relationship. Now, a role relationship can be very personal, but it has rather clear limits: some kinds of actions and attitudes fit within it, some are misfits. A parent's relation to her child is a highly personal one, and yet it would seem odd if a mature woman confided her inner fears and doubts to her teen-aged daughter and turned to her for consolation. A high school teacher may form a very personal rapport with his students, but were he to spend his evenings and weekends hanging around with them, the students themselves would feel something was wrong with him. The nurse relates to her patient within such a role, basically a role of caring. She needs the quality of availability—the ability to understand and accept her patient as he is, as a unique person. But she can't really expect to find such acceptance for herself—though that may happen, and then her patient may become her friend. She needs to understand and sympathize with her patient's fears and suffering, but *within the relationship of caring*, to console and to heal the suffering, rather than to share it. The young nurse whose patient became upset before surgery needed to learn to control her own response to fit the patient's need rather than letting her feelings match her patient's or trying to suppress her feelings altogether.

So the nurse's relationship with her patient needs to be involved and personal, though not an emotional identification with the patient. And at the same time that relationship needs to be detached and objective, though not cold and impersonal.

But there are needs a patient has that the nurse is helpless to meet and sufferings she is helpless to console. A patient cries out in severe pain that for some reason cannot be alleviated, and the nurse feels a knot of frustration because for all her caring there is nothing she can do for him. A patient trembles in fear of dying, and the nurse painfully realizes how empty words can be. A young patient in whose struggle for life she has been a watchful and caring partner begins to decline despite her intense efforts and prayers, and she watches helplessly as life departs. Her mind resounds with the question her tight and dry tongue could not form, why, why, why? And for her too there is no answer to that question, Job's question. There is only the silent darkness that marks the boundary of the human condition. And if she is to go on, without her capacity genuinely to care scorched and parched (she is told, you musn't let these things get to you), she needs the same stark faith that was Job's too. God is there in that darkness, her patient is in God's hands; she is too, in her very helplessness. She needs to let go, to trust herself and her patient to the hands of God. Then she will be free to care to the utmost limit of her ability, and yet be at peace when that limit is passed.

Within her relationship with her patients, the nurse is challenged to develop a subtle sensitivity to inner needs, a kind of sixth sense to discern a profound need among the routine requirements of care, to recognize an unspoken call for help and deep availability among a hundred greetings and requests. An apparently pointless conversation about the weather may conceal a very pointed, though unconscious, question: will you stop to listen to me? Will you recognize and care for me as a person?

The nurse who cares for seriously ill and dying patients has a particular need for such sensitivity. She has a hundred tasks to do—routine patient care, paperwork, responding to calls, more paperwork. A patient says in an offhand way, "nurse, got a minute?" If her mind is filled with her own business, the nurse may in effect answer "No." But if she is alert, she might realize a dying patient's need to talk about death, and as well his deep-rooted reluctance to bring such thoughts to the surface. "Got a minute?" may well mean that this is *the* moment when his anxiety and need are great enough to overcome the reluctance, and that out of all the people in this patient's world she is the one to whom he turns. For him the time is *now*. The nurse's business can wait. One nurse told of a particularly busy day, and a terminal patient whose condition was apparently stable called to her just when she was busiest. "I'll stop by in a few minutes," she said. When she returned, he was gone. Now she advises other nurses to drop *everything* and listen, unless doing so would actually jeopardize the life of another patient.

Of course there are mistakes and there are failures, and the nurse may be burdened with a sense of guilt, especially if she has an experience like the one described above. These mistakes and failures—of course, assuming they are not due to negligence or incompetence—confront the nurse with her own limitation as a human being. The guilt she feels warns her against becoming too self confident, too complacent. But if it is not to paralyze her, she needs again to let go, to trust herself and her patients to the hands of God. Then she will be free to care to the limit of her ability, and be able to accept herself— perhaps with a gentle sense of humor—when that limit is passed.

Patients And Their Families Are People

The nostalgic picture of bygone days when life was simpler (if indeed there was a time when life was simple in the living of it) includes an image of a warm personal relationship between folksy family doctors and their patients. But in the years following World War II, the developing specialization within the medical profession, the gradual coming of the doctor shortage, and the increasing complexity of hospital care changed that image. Each doctor served more and more patients. Often instead of one doctor there was a team of specialists, each caring for an aspect of the patient—so that the patient himself as a whole person began to feel forgotten. Larger hospitals performed more complex tasks for more people, but in order to do so they tended to stress efficiency and orderly routine over individualized care. As a result of these and similar developments, there arose a real danger of depersonalizing medical care, of forgetting that the patient is a person and not just a subject of treatment. Alert to that danger, some concerned medical professionals spoke out as early as 1950, calling for a more humanistic approach to patient care and to medical training. But the danger persists— and it is significant to note that systematic efforts to take the humanity of patients fully into account are still considered to be innovative. Fortunately, though, more and more medical professionals, especially nurses, are doing what they can to relate to their patients as people.

As persons, patients and their families need to be given a responsible role in health care. They need to be adequately informed about their illness and the plan of care. And when possible they appreciate the opportunity to contribute directly to their care.

But unless the doctor, the hospital and its staff take special care to meet these needs, the patient and especially his family may find themselves virtually ignored as persons. His family may find that the doctor is too busy really to talk with them. They may turn to the hospital's counseling service only to find that little specific information is available. Inevitably they turn to the nurse.

The nurse is in a position to listen to patient and family, answer questions, inform them—within limits—about the patient's care, and to provide opportunities for responsible participation in his care. And she may find all that and more demanded of her. So she may become resentful, looking on the questions and requests of patient and family as obstacles put in her way, preventing her from carrying out her duties efficiently. But such resentment betrays a failure to recognize her patients as people. If on the other hand she is able to look at the situation from their point of view, to step for a moment into their world of worry and confusion, she can make a decisive difference for them.

First, she can provide them with information, telling patient and family the reasons behind the patient's regimen, to an extent the nature and purpose of his medication, and ways they can cooperate and aid in the process of care. Here the nurse who has spent years studying will find her background in science especially valuable.

The nurse can provide opportunities for decision making on the part of the patient and family. More and more nurses try to develop a sort of contract relationship with their patients, allowing the patient some significant sense of choice. The routine schedule of care can be worked out and agreed upon between patient and nurse, rather than being imposed. Instead of simply performing her tasks, she can explain them, give the patient opportunity to question, and call for his approval. In this way the patient gains some sense of responsibility for himself, and he feels less like a thing crammed into a mechanical structure.

The nurse may be able to provide opportunities for a patient's family to participate in his care. Even simply washing the patient may mean for a spouse the difference between sitting helplessly like an outsider and having a sense of really contributing to the patient's well-being. There are many such tasks that, given instruction and some supervision, family members can perform effectively and with a sense of satisfaction.

Mindful that patients are people, the medical professional can foster a quality of relationships that can greatly help the effort to care. Providing complete information to patient and family develops a relationship of trust and confidence. So for instance the time it takes a nurse to provide such information may be more than made up by a decrease in the worried questions and requests that come from concerned people who are left helpless in their own care. Responsibility for decisions and for participation in the program of care develops a relationship of cooperation, so that a patient's family members—far from being a hindrance—can become effective partners of the medical professionals.

The effort to respect patients as people may also help to avoid some problems that can seriously hamper care. The person who is kept in a position of dependence, given little or no responsibility, may respond by a kind of regression into childish attitudes, including peevishness and stubbornness. Or he may even respond by trying to thwart the effort to care for him, finding a kind of satisfaction born of resentment in causing the medical professionals to fail and then expressing his resentment in bitter complaining.

If medical professionals forget that patients and their families are people, they can intensify the sense of helplessness, isolation and alienation that is already enough of a burden from the mere fact of being sick, and they can even undo their own efforts to care. But if they keep in mind the human dimension of caring, their patients and they themselves will be the healthier for it.

Concern for patients as persons is an ongoing concern for the health care professions and institutions. A recent expression of that concern is a "Patient's Bill of Rights" issued by the American Hospital Association in November, 1972. While it is not quite a binding law, it does state a set of assumptions about the relationship of medical professionals to patients, and it acts as a reminder that patients are people. The bill is summarized in an article in the September-October 1973 issue of *Society*:

1. The patient has the right to considerate and respectful care.

2. The patient has the right to obtain from his physician complete current information concerning his diagnosis, treatment and prognosis in terms the patient can reasonably be expected to understand.

3. The patient has the right to receive from his physician information necessary to give informed consent prior to the start of any procedure and/or treatment.

4. The patient has the right to refuse treatment to the extent permitted by law, and to be informed of the medical consequences of his action.

5. The patient has the right to every consideration of his privacy concerning his own medical care program.

6. The patient has the right to expect that all communications and records pertaining to his care should be treated as confidential.

7. The patient has the right to expect that within its capacity a hospital must make reasonable response to the request of the patient for services.

8. The patient has the right to obtain information as to any relationship of his hospital to other health care and educational institutions insofar as his care is concerned.

9. The patient has the right to be advised if the hospital proposes to engage in or perform human experimentation affecting his care or treatment.

10. The patient has the right to expect reasonable continuity of care.

11. The patient has the right to examine and receive an explanation of his bill regardless of source of payment.

12. The patient has the right to know what hospital rules and regulations apply to his conduct as a patient.

Efforts like this remind patients, families, and medical professionals of the simplest but most important aspect of health care, that in all its complexity it is people doing their best to care for people.

Chapter 8

Facing Ethical Challenges

A quick look through the literature on medical ethics would tell a person two things about this field. The first is that it is vast, touching on questions from the professional relationships among doctors to the much-publicized issues of abortion and euthanasia. The second is that to many of the questions raised in medical ethics there are no ready answers.

But the reality that medical ethics describes is a very specific one—it is people making decisions that affect the lives of other people. The vast extent of the field indicates that there are many people who must make many decisions. And the lack of ready answers indicates that very many of those decisions are difficult, indeed filled with uncertainty, conflict, and anguish.

So perhaps the basic question that needs to be asked in medical ethics is the fundamental question of all ethics: how does a person go about making an ethically good decision? How does a person go about making a truly responsible ethical judgment?

Our first concern will be to examine the nature and difficulty of responsible judgment in the face of a challenging ethical situation. The kind of situation that is most likely to present such a problem is currently that of the care of the dying: as medical technology has developed better techniques and equipment for saving the lives of people, the problem of "pulling the plug," or withdrawing life-support equipment when a patient is considered beyond saving, has become a particularly acute one. Then we will turn our attention to a problem that deserves special consideration from the point of view we have been taking—the problem of telling the truth about their condition to patients who are dying.

A Challenge To Responsible Decision

There is a certain kind of moral training which stresses rather clear-cut do's and (especially) don'ts, and no doubt many people who have grown up within a Christian family and especially who have gone through church schools have been trained in this way, trained to expect moral and ethical problems to be rather clear and straightforward. One does not steal. This act would be stealing. Therefore one should not do it. This way of thinking and of living serves quite well for many people most of the time, providing a clear sense of right and wrong and a tool for organizing one's moral life in a reliable way.

But there are times when a person is presented with a challenge that forces him to rethink this clear-cut, straightforward morality. For it is easy to see what is right and what is wrong when right and wrong stand apart as if on display, appropriately classified and labeled. But real moral challenges never come so neatly packaged. Questions that might seem clear in the thinking of them become cloudy in the living of them, for they never occur alone, but always as part of a situation complicated by many other considerations, some of them other ethical questions of equal weight. An ethical decision in such a situation is not a matter of "doing the right thing"—it is a matter of trying to make the best of a dilemma. That killing is wrong, for instance, seems clear enough in the ten commandments. But what happens to that clear-cut commandment not to kill when a person is a soldier in a war? A policeman confronting a man who may be armed?

In such times, in such situations, a person is called upon to make a responsible judgment. There is no answer that is completely right. And whatever decision is made, especially if it is one involving a person's life, the one who makes the decision has to live with the clear realization that it could have been otherwise, and that he is responsible. And so the call to responsible ethical judgment can bring pain and anguish with it. Our concern includes then not only the nature of responsible judgment, but the meaning of the anguish it brings with it.

A situation to consider

The decision to continue or to stop life support treatment for the hopelessly terminal patient is a particularly difficult one. The anguish of that kind of decision is especially acute for the persons closest to the patient: his family first, but in a very important way the nurse or nurses who have cared for him.

Mr. Y, a man in his early thirties, had entered the hospital for treatment of a recurring ear infection. He was the father of two young children, and except for the infection enjoyed good health. A few days after his admission he showed symptoms of meningitis. He worsened in spite of antibiotics and went into a coma, and so was transferred for care to the Intensive Care Unit of the hospital. The very day he was brought to the ICU, he showed signs of irreversible brain damage: he did not respond to painful stimuli, the pupils of his eyes were dilated and fixed, and he had other abnormal neurological responses. Nevertheless, special treatment was initiated to bring the antibiotics directly to the surface of his brain. His breathing stopped two days after he entered the ICU, but he was put on a respirator. A further special treatment was then initiated to bathe his spinal column with antibiotics. It was another full week before his family was told that he would not recover. He finally died after two full weeks in the ICU. Those two weeks meant a time of intense uncertainty and pain for his family, and they meant financial ruin as well. At the same time for the doctors and nurses who cared for him it could be considered a period of heroic struggle to save his life.

Things need not have gone that way. What actually happened was the result of decisions which could well have

been different. And what actually happened could be interpreted in different ways by the different people involved.
Some insight into the nature and difficulty of responsible
judgment can be gained by looking closely at those decisions
from the point of view of the medical professional, especially
the nurse, and from the point of view of the family of the
patient.

Some general guidelines and problems

At several points in Mr. Y's illness a decision could have
been made to stop further treatment. Irreversible brain
damage was evident on the day of his entry into the ICU. At
the time of his breathing failure it was evident that his vital
functions could not continue unless sustained by the respirator. His lack of progress from that point on indicated the
probable futility of the efforts to save him.

But such a decision is not lightly reached, for it is a decision
involving a person's life—and as well the integrity of the
medical profession. Persons who face such a decision seek
guidelines to help them be as just and objective as possible in
the situation.

One guideline goes back to the distinction made by Pope
Pius XII between the ordinary means of preserving life and
extraordinary means. There is an obligation to work to save a
person's life within the limits of the ordinary methods of care,
but extraordinary treatment, equipment, or risks are not
morally necessary—though they may be freely chosen by
patient or family with the doctor's advice. The problem with
this distinction is that what is ordinary and what is extraordinary is not all that clear. Machinery and medication that
today is quite customary was unheard of in the late forties,
when Pius XII proposed this guideline. And so the doctor and
family find themselves facing a further decision: whether a
proposed treatment is ordinary or extraordinary is to an
extent a matter of judgment. A workable guide to judgment
here is offered by Professor Paul Ramsey: "ordinary means"
would be medication or treatment which can offer a reason-

able hope of benefit without excessive pain, expense, or inconvenience. So, for instance, an experimental operation with only a slim chance of success need not be performed, or at least one need not sense any moral obligation to perform or consent to such an operation.

A second guideline sought is a clear understanding of when death occurs. It once was enough to say that a person was dead when his breathing and heart stopped. But recent developments have made it possible to revive a person in that condition. Some current efforts to redefine death have developed the notion of death as "brain death"—indicated by a flat electroencephalogram taken at least twice over a period of twenty-four hours. This might occur even though other vital functions are still being maintained with the help of life-support machinery. One important application of such a definition would be in the situation when another patient is in need of a vital organ for a transplant: but in this case, the twenty-four hour period called for to protect the dying patient from premature death becomes a serious problem for another whose life might be saved if a transplant can be performed in time. And so the attempt to define death confronts a new dilemma. A further difficulty that would remain even if a clear legal definition of death was achieved is the gap that exists between definitions and reality. The difference between death and life according to the definition might be scarcely perceptible to one who is observing the dying patient—and the application of the definition might itself seem a matter of a decision rather than a simple perception of the obvious.

Two problems arise to complicate the dilemma of those who must decide. The first is a marked tendency on the part of some medical professionals to deny the inevitability of a patient's death. This is understandable, considering that a doctor's entire preparation is oriented toward the maintaining of life and the restoration of health. No doctor likes to lose a patient even if death is inevitable, and so he may fight the discouraging diagnosis until he finds not the slightest hope, and even then he may not share with the nurse and especially with the patient or family his conviction that the disease is terminal. A result of this tendency is the agonizing delay that we saw before Mr. Y's family was informed that he was indeed dying.

Another problem, perhaps a danger, is a tendency among a few medical professionals to figure that if a patient is terminal, there is no sense in doing anything more for him. In some cases this tendency results in patients with a long-term illness like cancer being left in the background as far as care is concerned, so that discomforts and even new ailments that arise may not be promptly or effectively cared for. And in a few cases this tendency results in actions which directly or indirectly hasten the death of a patient. It is this danger—euthanasia—which may prompt hesitation on the part of the conscientious medical professional to withdraw life-support systems from a patient like Mr. Y.

The dilemma of the nurse

The nurse finds herself in a paradoxical position in regard to the decision to "pull the plug" or not. Most significant for her is that she is generally not in a position to participate in the decision, for it is usually made by the patient's family and doctor. And yet in many ways she is more fully aware of the total situation than doctor or family. As a medical professional who has the responsibility for carrying out the care of the patient, she is aware of his condition and prognosis. She is also likely to have gotten to know the family and their situation, and so to have an understanding of the impact of the illness on them emotionally and financially. And whatever decision is made, she will be the one to carry out its particulars. If life-support is to be continued, she is the one who has the responsibility of maintaining it. And if it is to be stopped, it is she who faces the concrete act of removing the tubes that have sustained the patient, of "pulling the plug."

The nurse then is likely to recognize the need for decision, and yet be unable to act herself. She meets obstacles whichever way she feels the decision should go. Here is a man whose life is at stake, and she wants to do all in her power to save him. As a medical professional, she knows what it is possible to do, especially with the techniques and equipment available in most urban hospitals. But before she can act to save life, as she has been prepared to do and as her whole vocation is oriented, she may have to wait for the approval—or disapproval—of the family. One young nurse complained that "those people are preventing us from saving life!" On the other hand, the nurse may be aware of the futility of further treatment and the emotional and financial havoc wrought in the family, and yet be bound by orders from a doctor who apparently fails to admit the obvious.

What can she do? The possibilities open to her for action vary with the situation in which she works. Ideally, since she is an educated medical professional, especially if she has had the advantage of a collegiate nursing program, she should be considered a member of the care-giving team. And so ideally she should have some input into the decision. But practically, she finds herself working within narrower limits. She can consult or discuss with the doctor about his feelings and values in relation to continuing life-support treatment, and can call his attention to the facts of the patient's current condition or share the observations she has been able to make as she works closely with the patient. And with the doctor's approval she can inform the family of the nature of his treatment, its chances of success, its expense, and the alternatives open to them. Here she has to be careful not to impose her own feelings on the family, especially anything that would arouse a feeling of guilt in them should they decide to discontinue life-support.

These are the problems and possibilities that she has. And so in a case like that of Mr. Y, she is in a position to balance the likelihood of real benefit from continued care against the burden placed on the family. And though she is not in a position to make the final decision, she herself does face a decision—whether to go along with the treatment unquestion-

ingly, or to raise the issue of "pulling the plug" with the doctor.

The family's dilemma

For the family of a dying person, the decision to maintain
or discontinue life-support treatment is filled with anguish. To
them this is not a "case," it is a person they love. Nevertheless,
they need to gain a certain objectivity if they are to make a
responsible decision. Perhaps achieving that objectivity is the
most challenging part of the problem.

The family faces obstacles to objectivity within themselves
and outside themselves. Within themselves first is the difficult
challenge of accepting the inevitable death of someone they
love. For unless they can recognize, admit, and accept the fact
of impending death, they may cling with irrational hope even
to medical procedures that provide very little real possibility
of success. And so they may be led by their own denial of
death into fruitless emotional and financial sacrifice. If they
accept the death of their loved one as a very real possibility,
they may be better able to consider the alternatives that are
open to them, including "pulling the plug," on their objective
merits.

There may also be within the family the temptation to give
in to guilt feelings. They may feel that they have failed the sick
person in some way—failed to appreciate him, disappointed
him, or caused him unhappiness in his healthier days. And
this feeling of guilt can express itself in an urge to sacrifice all
in life saving effort that is at best chancy, and most likely
futile. Another source of guilt may be the family's sense of
what is expected in such a situation, perhaps an attitude of
noblesse oblige. A family member might ask what others have
done in similar circumstances, and feel an obligation to
continue life-support treatment at all costs if others had
chosen to do so. Or instead of looking at the alternatives fully
and objectively, someone might beg the question by phrasing
them as "trying to save his life" as against "just letting him

die." In this regard, doctors and nurses need to be a bit cautious in the way they present the situation to the family, for they might unwittingly reinforce such guilt feelings and so impair the family's ability to judge objectivity.

In such cases, the patient himself may have provided his family with an aid to objective judgment. An increasing number of people are making out what is called a "Living Will," which states the desire that if sudden fatal illness or accident strikes, they be allowed to "die with dignity" without unusual or expensive treatment that has little certainty of success. Such a statement suggests a calm acceptance of death and counsels objectivity in those who must make the decision, without closing the door to responsible efforts to save life.

The family may meet an obstacle to responsible judgment outside themselves, for the doctor may withhold from them the kind of information they need. In Mr. Y's case, the family was not told clearly of his condition until difficult and costly treatment had already been given for a week and a half. Fortunately the family is called upon to sign a form consenting to treatment, but often they are asked in effect to sign a blank check, consenting to any and all procedures the doctor deems useful. Or if the specific procedure is proposed for their consent, they are often left in ignorance about its specific nature, its cost and its chances of success. In effect, their choice is blindly to trust the doctor or coldly to let the patient die. So they can be deprived of the opportunity for truly responsible decision.

Judgment

In Mr. Y's case, there were several points along the way which called for responsible decision, each of them slightly more clear and less ambiguous. Unfortunately the family was not fully informed of his condition until rather late, and so the decision was made by the doctor.

When he did not respond to the usual treatment for meningitis, a decision was made to bring him to the ICU for specialized treatment. Should this have been done? For doctor and nurse, the alternatives were rather clear: it appeared that Mr. Y could be restored to health if he received the treatment. To deny him the treatment would in effect contradict their responsibility as persons dedicated to the maintaining of life and the restoration of health.

On that same day, he showed clear signs of irreversible brain damage. There was no move to discontinue the treatment, but the alternatives were significantly changed. Now the best that could be hoped for was a greatly reduced life—Mr. Y might survive, but he would never regain consciousness. And now the likelihood of his survival was also significantly reduced. And yet the treatment was continued for two more weeks. At this point the family could have been alerted—and in fact the "Patient's Bill of Rights" would indicate that they should have been kept informed of Mr. Y's condition even before this point and now allowed to exercise the right to refuse treatment. But they were not.

What could a nurse in this situation do? She could have acted to raise the question of discontinuing treatment with the doctor. To have done so, though, given the particular hospital structure in which she found herself, to speak out could mean taking a risk of reprimand with little assurance that anything would be done to alert the family. She chose not to act, and treatment was continued.

When Mr. Y's breathing failed and he had to be maintained by a respirator, the alternatives were again changed. Now even an unconscious existence was not likely without the aid of expensive life-support equipment, though a small chance remained that his condition might be stabilized at the level of unconscious existence. Again a point of decision was reached and passed without informing the family and giving them the opportunity for judgment. And yet the doctor chose to struggle further to preserve such reduced life. Now, were that the only value to be considered—the preservation of life—he might well go on without hesitation. But every day of this treatment was costing Mr. Y's young family dearly, both financially and emotionally. And if the treatment were to succeed in saving this life, the most optimistic concrete result short of a miracle would be that Mr. Y's family would be given the burden of caring indefinitely for a hopelessly unconscious person. Granted that such a burden can have profound meaning for those who bear it, imposing such a burden is as serious a consideration as permitting the disease to take its course. Especially at this point, it would be irresponsible for the doctor to ignore that side of the situation. And yet even further new treatments were ordered and continued for another full week before the family was advised that he would not live. And then they were put in the position of having to accept the inevitable rather than given the opportunity for responsible judgment.

But what if they had been given that opportunity at the point when Mr. Y showed irreversible brain damage? Or at the point when his breathing failed? If they were able to consider the situation objectively, they would be called upon to weigh the probable benefit of further treatment against the burden it presented in its present cost and in the projected need for continuous care. It would be important for them to realize that by the time his illness had progressed to such a point where his life could not be saved without treatment that can reasonably be considered extraordinary, there would be no clear obligation to continue the treatment. The option would be open—with no clear do's and don'ts, but only the call for intelligent and responsible decision.

Anguish

One of the most difficult aspects of a real moral challenge— one demanding responsible judgment in the face of a dilemma rather than being a clear-cut matter—is that there is no reassuring sense of being justified in one's action. Whichever way a decision would be made in relation to Mr. Y, those who are responsible for the decision know that it could well be otherwise. And so they may well feel uneasy, even guilty.

For the nurse, even though her role in the decision is indirect, there is a particularly direct anguish if treatment is discontinued. For to her falls the task of actually removing the life-support equipment. And as she does so, no matter how hopeless the patient's prognosis, she realizes that her action removes all ambiguity: this is the end. And she can't help wondering if perhaps in another day unforeseen developments would have saved the patient. Though the decision is made by others, her action means the concrete end of hope, no matter how slender. And so in a way it is easier to carry on the "heroic struggle," for that provides a reassuring sense of having done what is right—unless, of course, the nurse is perceptive enough to see the emotional ravages worked on the family and to sense their despair at their financial situation. If she is so perceptive, or perhaps we can say morally sensitive, then her lot is anguish whichever way the decision goes.

For the family, no matter how hopeless the patient's situation, the decision to discontinue treatment means decision that yes, he shall die now. There is a guilt, a fear—irrational perhaps but real—that they are responsible for their loved one's death, as if that were under their control. They fear that they have played God, or that they have failed to give God a chance—as if they might expect some sort of miracle. And so for the family, too, it is in a way easier to go the way of heroic sacrifice, suffering hardship for a long period in order to avoid such a reproach. But if they are perceptive, morally sensitive to their own motivation, they may realize that the struggle and the hardship were the price not of life but of self-justification—something fundamentally selfish, though in a subtle way.

The significance of a real moral challenge and the anguish that it brings can be sought precisely in the frustration of a person's desire to feel justified in his action. He has made a decision, and he has no way of knowing if it was "right"—or even what the word "right" means in relation to it. He has to live with that decision, and with its ambiguity.

Perhaps there is a clue to that significance in an enigmatic statement Jesus made to the Pharisees who criticized him for associating with people who weren't considered "respectable."

He said "It is not those who are well who need the doctor, but
the sick. I have not come to call the virtuous, but sinners to
repentance." (Luke 5:31–32). There is a great distance between being virtuous, having the feeling that one always does
the "right" thing, and living the Christian life. Christianity,
after all, is not a process of self-justification; it is not a way of
virtue that leads a man to feel good about himself. It is a way
of repentance—of self-*denial*. It is a call to give up the futile
attempt to justify oneself and to accept an undeserved relationship with God which is freely offered to him in Christ.
Yes, there are feelings of guilt. Yes, there is anguish. Yes,
there is frustration at having no way to turn that is clearly in
the right. But that is what it means to be a finite human being
whose meaning is not quite under his control. That is what it
means to be called to faith in God. For to the morally honest
person, there is no unambiguous assurance that he is right: he
relies not on his own virtue but on the grace of God. For him,
the anguish of a real moral challenge can be a call to deeper
faith.

Responsible ethical judgment, then, involves two basic
dimensions. The first is understanding the various aspects of
the challenging situation in as fair and objective a way as
possible. This means taking into account whatever guidelines
are available and judiciously applying them to the situation;
examining the real values involved—in Mr. Y's case, his life,
the integrity of the medical profession, and the welfare of his
family; and estimating as well as possible the consequences of
alternate courses of action. The second is simply decision—
stepping beyond everything that is generally defined and
everything that is ambiguous and making a specific choice,
taking a specific action. This means the anguish of uncertainty and the renunciation of the illusory assurance that one
is doing the "right thing."

To Tell Or Not To Tell

A person reflecting as a Christian on the problems and
challenges facing the sick and dying discovers from time to

time practices and attitudes that contradict and frustrate the call to faith and to spiritual depth that sickness can mean. One such practice is the distressingly common reluctance of medical professionals to tell a terminal patient that he is indeed dying. While this practice does not suggest the serious ethical disorder of the sort that is involved in, say, euthanasia, it does suggest a basic failure to take responsibly into account the religious and indeed humanistic dimension of sickness and dying.

It is distressing to discover that denial, the deliberate effort to conceal from a terminal patient the fact that he is dying, is practiced by a majority of physicians. Estimates of the number of doctors who habitually practice denial range from 60% to 95%. Of course many of those who conceal the truth from a patient may inform the nurse, and eventually the family—but often with the directive that the patient himself is not to learn of it.

One rationale for this practice is based on an interesting notion of "appropriate death." A peaceful death without upset, without anxiety, and especially without any disturbance of hospital routine is an appropriate death. Values to be achieved are comfort for the patient, as high a level of present activity and interest as possible until the end, and the avoidance of any confrontation with words or procedures that suggest death. Dangers to be avoided are risks of emotional outbursts that would be stressful to the patient and disturbing to others, and depression, which might hasten death. And the best way to avoid these dangers is to prevent the patient from the explicit knowledge that he is dying.

The difficulty with this line of thought is that it bases its entire judgment on the external, the observable. Granted, the intangible spiritual process of dying we probed earlier does not respond to scientific methods of measurement, and indeed is scoffed at by some behaviorally oriented thinkers. But a very serious question must be raised in the face of this line of thought, and in the name of the dying patient as a person with an interior life, a spiritual destiny that is very much at stake in this critical act of dying.

Within the limits of scientific observation, there may be no evidence for what we have called the mystery of dying. But to proceed from a lack of evidence to the practical denial of a reality is highly unscientific. For there is no evidence, nor is empirical or behavioral evidence possible, which can provide the slightest support for the *non*existence of a death-transcending reality in man. And so an authentically scientific attitude would call for an openness here: at least allowing for the real possibility of an interior life and a spiritual destiny. To act without taking that possibility into account—and positively to make a terminal patient avoid confrontation with death is to act without taking it into account—is to act irresponsibly.

Perhaps, though, the practice of denial is not in most cases quite as deliberate as that. There may be another rationale, unspoken, that leads a doctor to conceal the truth from his patient. He voices a fear of upsetting the patient. But two questions might lead us to wonder if the real reason is another fear. First, there are ways to tell the patient—perhaps with much preparation and tact—which minimize the danger of upset. So the doctor's fear should be directed not at the telling itself but at the manner of telling. Second, if denial is so prevalent a practice, then a very high percentage of terminal patients must give the doctor reason to fear they will respond to the truth in a highly emotional way. We might wonder that there is not a greater variety among terminal patients. But our wondering may well turn back toward the doctor himself. After all, he has been trained to save life, and his whole vocation is that of a healer. In the face of death he is powerless, and he may consider himself defeated. Perhaps the one who is upset is the doctor, and to tell his patient that death is inevitable may be as difficult for him as a confession of failure. Such a concern and fear is surely understandable, and it is easy to sympathize with the doctor. But the ethical problem involved is that the spiritual welfare of the patient is apparently being disregarded, and the doctor may well be acting out of a disguised concern for himself, or at least an unreflected taking of the path that is easiest for him rather than ultimately best for the patient.

The result of denial can be serious for the patient and his family. Were he aware of his impending death, he would have the opportunity to prepare himself for it. One aspect of that preparation might be setting his affairs in order for the good of his family. Here a consequence of denial could be a costly legal tangle that would be avoided if the dying person had the opportunity to make or alter his will. But the spiritual aspect of the patient's preparation for death is of ultimate importance. Yes, a period of upset might well occur, but that is one stage that a person may go through in his struggle to meet the challenge of dying. He is not to be prevented from facing it; he is to be helped through it. If he is kept from knowing his prognosis in advance, he faces the full challenge of death in a briefer, more desperate time when death is so close it is obvious to him. Placing a patient in that situation is like sending a green soldier into the thick of battle with no time for training.

A Christian and even a humanistic approach of the care of the dying would call for a change in this practice of fostering denial. And in fact a merely legal approach would indicate it is no longer possible to maintain the practice of denial, for patients now have the legal right to see their medical charts and to have the basic information on those charts accurately interpreted to them, within limits.

Would we say then that a terminal patient should simply be told flatly of his terminal status as soon as it is known? Hardly—such an approach would amount to a kind of violent disregard for the emotional needs of the patient as person. Again, what is called for is not a clear-cut universal policy, but a responsible judgment in a difficult and ambiguous situation.

The positive effort to prepare a patient to die is unfortunately rather rare. A certain hesitancy to turn from physiological to religious concerns, and a reluctance to deal with death as a simple reality of life seem to characterize many who are charged with the care of the dying. And such hesitancy and reluctance is understandable, for it is not an easy thing to accept the reality of death, even in another person.

And so what is called for is not a simple change of behavior, but a complex change of attitude and values. Fortunately, signs of such change are evident. The cosmetic complex used to hide the reality of death in our society seems to be melting away, as more and more educators, social scientists, theologians, and doctors take a good look at death and seek to understand it. Discussions of death and dying are introduced into the training of nurses. And patients and their families are becoming more frank in their questions and concerns. The basic change that is needed is for those who care for the dying to come to terms with the reality of death themselves.

With such a recognition and acceptance as a basis, perhaps it is possible to develop a sensitive yet honest approach to preparing terminal patients for dying. Those caring for him should be honest, and so truth should be the value governing their dealing with the patient. Yet they should be sensitive, bringing each patient gently to recognize the truth of his condition and realistically and hopefully to prepare. Perhaps many, if not most terminal patients, would not be able to stand a blunt revelation that they were about to die. Perhaps upset or depression would follow. But that does not mean that the truth should be kept from them. Rather it means that they need to be prepared and guided to the point where they can recognize and accept death. For that is something they are unavoidably called to do anyway: to persist in denial spares them no pain, it simply spares those caring for them a certain amount of inconvenience and effort.

But how and when and by whom they should be guided toward the truth will depend entirely on the character of the patient and on the kinds of relationships he has with family and others who care for him. The success of those efforts to guide is by no means guaranteed, though what the patient expresses and what he thinks and feels within him may be quite different things.

Unsolicited false assurances from the doctor can readily be avoided, and it is these that sound most suspiciously as if they are addressed to the doctor himself. Flat lies in response to questions of the patient can be quite dangerous, for it is quite possible that the patient suspects the truth, and denial in the face of a direct question endangers the trust that is needed between patient and those who care for him. But a direct question is not necessarily seeking an answer. Perhaps it is seeking a caring response, the availability of a human being in a critical time. The patient can be allowed to speak the fear or worry that he has, and if his fears are true then there is little real purpose in denying them. And yet to say "Yes, it's incurable cancer, you're going to die" can be brutal. The truth can be conveyed gently with a nod, a firm holding of a hand, the honest assurance that "we'll do all we can to make you comfortable." If beneath the response is a recognition and respect for the mystery of dying that this person is facing, perhaps the simplest gesture can communicate valuable strength.

Here there are no clear-cut do's and don'ts, there is only the call to responsible judgment. Here the basic reality is not guidelines or practices, but caring persons acting out of a concern for the patient as a person with an inner life and a death-transcending destiny.

Part IV

Some Special Challenges

Three forms of sickness are singled out for particular reflection because they add special dimensions to its call. Aging is special because it is not exactly an illness, though it brings with it many of the sufferings of sickness. The handicapped are special because they must learn to live in a world which too often fails to accept them as persons. And mental illness is special because most often it is not a physical ailment but a suffering that attacks the very personality.

Chapter 9

A Way Of Aging

As a person grows to the age when his grandchildren are about as tall as he, when he has more than enough time to do all the fishing, reading, puttering and maybe traveling that for years he'd promised himself, but maybe hasn't quite got the energy to go and actually do it all, he may sense a certain frustration and disappointment. He may discover that in some ways his experience is like that of the seriously sick person. The activities that once filled his day and the concerns that once filled his mind become remote, and with them the people with whom he shared them. He finds his powers increasingly limited. And he may find himself more and more alone. But there is a significant difference for the aging person: he may be perfectly healthy! He doesn't experience his condition as an interruption in his life, a temporary situation from which he hopes to return to "normal." Aging is perfectly normal, not an interruption. And there is no return from it. Further, the aging person is not singled out for exceptional suffering—he can hardly ask "why me?" He knows that he walks in the way of all humanity.

And so the challenge that faces the healthy aging person is a special one—in some ways analogous to the challenge of sickness, and in some ways unique. And the successful facing of that challenge can produce in a person a quality often associated with "the elders": wisdom. The way of aging can be a way to wisdom.

Problems and Disappointments

There is an interesting twist to the pursuit of paradise that is so characteristic of our American culture. Despite the apparent ease of access people have to the trappings of paradise—happiness advertised in packs of twenty, success in a bonded bottle or (to up the ante) in an amply chromed automobile, ecstacy in a luxurious vacation shangri-la—for most people these things are far beyond immediate reach. And so we are schooled in the virtue of "delayed gratification"—work hard now, be frugal, sacrifice, but look ahead to the day when your efforts will pay off a hundredfold in your own private earthly paradise. The young man looks forward to the day he will "arrive," the established family looks forward to the day when their burdens and expenses will decrease instead of steadily increasing, and the middle-aged look forward to the day when they will be free of their burdens and have the leisure to enjoy the fruits of their labors: retirement. As long-awaited day approaches when the children are on their own and when the faithful worker has been given praises and maybe a gold watch as he is ceremoniously escorted to the exit door, a person has every right (according to the philosophy of the advertisement, anyway) to expect that door to be the entrance to a paradisal state, to the much-touted "golden years."

'Tain't necessarily so

It can be a rude awakening when the person who goes through that magic door discovers that it simply leads *out*, out of the entangling but fulfilling life of the family, and out of the burdensome but significant world of career and work. He has invested his life in a dream, and when he arrives at the awaited time, there is no substance to the dream. He is free of burdens and entanglements, yes. But free for what? He can now do anything he wants—but what is there worth wanting? He has gone through the door of what may have seemed at times a prison, but he discovers it leads nowhere but *out*—he no longer has a real place among his fellowmen, and no longer can sense just where he fits in.

In another age, in a society with a slower pace and steadier tradition than ours, the aging person might step into a significant and satisfying place. He would be regarded as a wise counselor, and his word would be weighty. But in our society he no longer counts, his word is considered obsolete, and he feels he is regarded almost with suspicion as a burden rather than a rich resource. He had found his identity in his work, but his work has turned him out at a specified age even though his capacities may not have decreased. His home and family had been his place, but now the children have grown, with lives of their own, and more than likely his spouse is no longer with him. His friends were either people he knew through his work or friends from youth. He loses contact with the first group when he leaves his work. And he sadly sees the circle of people he'd known for years shrinking as he finds himself more and more aware of the obituary column in the newspaper. He is *out*—and more and more alone, with no significant role to play any more.

He had been told that the treasures of leisure are now his. And he may have dreamed as a youth of having the time to travel, or to develop skill in art or handicrafts. However, he finds his curiosity about faraway places waning as he gains time to see them. Travel is an enriching education, he has told himself. But for what is he enriching himself? Why should he educate himself? What use is it to anybody, and what contribution can he make where he has no place any more? He discovers that art and handicrafts take a long-term effort if a person is going to do anything worthwhile in them. Making things is a joy, he has told himself. But in itself it is work, and unless his own appreciation is shared by others, the motivation for tedious effort is not likely to stay with him. The others he had dreamed would share the fruit of his work are changed now or gone—children now no longer children and not really interested in grampa's knickknacks. And so his dream may dwindle into a poignant regret that he hadn't done his traveling or developed his hobby earlier in life. Instead of holding the treasures of leisure he finds himself empty-handed, with time heavy and nothing of significance to do with himself.

He had been led to expect that age would bring with it a certain wisdom. But as he passed through the door that promised all these things, he felt no particular inspiration, and now folks younger than he tend to discount his opinions (he suspects maybe rightly sometimes, since education has become more common since he grew up). Wisdom hasn't come automatically, and he gets little enlightenment on where to look for it. Of course, "wisdom" is a word not that frequently used in our highly technical society, and may not be readily recognized among people who are susceptible to the advertised trappings of earthly paradise. Even the elder who has arrived at a sort of wisdom may find that the market for it is slow indeed.

And so it is not surprising if an aging person feels a certain frustration and disappointment, a sense that somehow he has been the victim in a subtle, intricate and all-embracing con game.

Left out

But even if his expectations were not so unrealistic, a number of factors combine to prevent a person from partici-pating as fully in life as he might like as he grows older.

He discovers—and it is no surprise, really—that there are some things he simply isn't physically capable of any more. He suddenly realizes it has been ten years or more since he has run. He thinks for a minute before lifting the heavy box or climbing the stairway that he wouldn't have blinked at in younger days. He finds he can't do without his sleep—and maybe a few extra winks in the lazy afternoon.

He soon discovers that he is subjected to subtle forms of prejudice. In a fast-moving, youth-oriented society, aging persons are often stereotyped. Graying hair is assumed to carry with it a whole complex of characteristics that are associated with old age, like extreme weakness, various diseases, and especially deteriorating mental powers. He is treated often with politeness, and sometimes with a rather patronizing manner that suggests to him that what he has to say and do is not being taken seriously. Further, he finds his leisure a handicap in a society where work and productivity tend to be the norms for defining a person's worth. Where a man feels he can come to know another man by asking what he does for a living, the retiree finds himself at a loss for an identity. He may have accomplished great things during his working years—but unless they have made him famous (enough so that the people he meets might have heard of them), no one is interested in what is past.

The aging person may find his confidence in himself slipping, partially because he recognizes a slowing of his powers, and partially because he half believes the stereotypes. For a man not to be working can mean for him a loss of his sense of worth, and for a woman whose family has been her life the departure of the children can leave her with no way of knowing her own value. And there is the fear that aging might bring senility with it, and the slightest lapse of memory or error in judgment—that would have passed without notice or with a laugh years earlier—now fills a person with worry and dismay. That very worry causes in turn a growing insecurity that produces increasing but really needless unsteadiness of thought and memory.

He learns too clearly that a "dynamic society" has a negative side—rapidly changing patterns of life and work leave him with a sense of being left behind the time, obsolete as a straight-eight automobile. And he suffers the dream-shattering erosion of his economic power because the dynamism of society is most often translated into steadily rising living costs, while his retirement income or his savings are likely to be fixed.

But most difficult of all is his recognition—that grows clearer with each day's obituary column—that the decline he senses is not a temporary condition, but the harbinger of death. Friends and acquaintances that are his contemporaries die. And where the death of a friend meant shock and sorrow years back, now it has a flavor of inevitability about it—oh, yes, now it is his turn, yes, I knew him when. . . . Unspoken is the realization that my turn is approaching too.

So the aging person finds himself left out of the mainstream of a society busy with the ever faster pursuit of paradise. He might well feel a certain irony in that. The forces that combine to exclude him are by-products of that frantic pursuit. And he has come to the bitter realization of its end result: like the chasing of the rainbow that recedes faster and faster one runs after it, the pursuit of the earthly paradise leads nowhere—for there is none. But were he to speak out that realization, the busy folk he speaks to would, he knows, smile, pat him on the head and say "Thanks," turn and say to each other "He's a sweet old man," and then charge headlong into the rush again.

Coping

A number of the problems that cause frustration to aging people seem to have ready solutions—or at least advertisers claim they have. Feel tired and weak? Just take a certain vitamin and iron supplement, and you'll stay in shape. All social awkwardness can be overcome by a truly effective denture adhesive. You can be "in" again if you buy into a recently (and hastily) constructed retirement village. And now there is Vitamin E. Rejoice: the pursuit of paradise is opened once again even to those old enough to know better!

And yet there are some realistic ways to cope with disappointments and problems, both those which are inevitable as a part of aging and those which are more frustrating because they are the result of misconceptions or prejudice. The attitude that a person takes toward his situation can make a big difference in its quality for him, and the kind of relationships a person is able to maintain can provide a sense of significance for him.

Acceptance

Perhaps the most basic attitude that can help a person is realistic acceptance of his condition. We have seen that even pain hurts less when it is accepted, and that the most confining situations can become in a way creative if a person embraces them with his whole person. A realistic acceptance means more than a steadfast effort to ignore the difficult side of things. Acceptance does not mean trying very hard to imagine that the "exit" door he went through actually did lead into a satisfying state. It means looking squarely at myself and my situation, seeing it for what it is—and then taking a creative stand in relation to it.

So I do feel a disappointment when I look at myself. No great dreams swell my ego as they did in youth—just some memories that aren't exactly impressive. And I finally have to admit that a lot of plans and projects just aren't ever going to be done. I look at myself now as I am, for what I've made of myself. And maybe for the first time I realize this is *me*—this, me, right here and now, no frills, no fancy ambitions—this. I seem pitifully small, now I haven't got a grandiose future as part of what I consider myself, the way a younger man has. But this is *really* me, and every last worn and maybe compromised bit of me is no dream, but real. Here I am, and being just what I am is what my whole life means right now. Being what I am, making no fancy claims.

There's a certain liberation, a kind of sigh of relief, in being able to say "this is me, that's all there is." It's not complacency, because it's not a feeling of self-satisfaction. There is a rueful quality—a sort of musing regret. The relief comes from not having to fuss and worry over making myself into some kind of ideal or career goal. But the liberation can be deeper than that.

Because there is a sense of *meaning* or *fulfillment* in such a realistic acceptance. I have my regrets, I feel a little rueful when I think of what I might have become were it not for what I am—but basically I don't hate myself. I can sense a kind of *affirmation*, a real sense of being happy with myself.

It's not that I tell myself I'm great in spite of everything. It's not that I make a sort of accounting of my good points and bad points and end up in the black. It's deeper, less artificial, and more real than that.

For if I look back over my life—the circumstances that kept me from doing some things I'd wanted, the unexpected opportunities that led me where I hadn't planned, people I've met, children who meant for me a challenge to love and a series of surprises—I get the very distinct idea that this unimpressive reality of me is not just the product of my own making. There was a guiding hand in it beyond mine—and that divine hand shaped me (though I might be stiff clay) at least as much as I shaped myself. So I sense an affirmation through the subtle presence of God in the simple reality of myself—ambiguous, there in spite of my failures or misguided wanderings, but real.

If a person can realistically accept himself in such a spirit of faith, that acceptance tends to bear fruit in other basic attitudes. For if such acceptance is present, then many frustrations—failing powers, prejudice, disappointed dreams —are reduced from frightening assaults on one's beseiged self-respect to real but incidental annoyances. They don't matter that much any more—so a person may be able to laugh at a lapse of memory or an error of judgment that might otherwise arouse considerable dismay. On the other hand, he will be able to appreciate and delight in what limited abilities and opportunities he has. So like the person facing a long hospital stay, he may find his sensitivity to the simple goods and beauties of life increasing, freed from the distraction of worriedly trying to be what he is not—or no longer is. So acceptance can give birth to a gentle ability to chuckle at oneself, to take oneself without too much seriousness. And that sense of humor flowers into a freedom from worry for oneself, and a freedom for delight in the simple reality of living in the world.

But acceptance bears a further fruit. For if I see myself for what I am, and come to sense the hand of God in what I have become—then I can as well sense that the hand of God is still there, forming, guiding and calling me. Yes, my grandiose future and my career ideals have evaporated back into the dreamland from which they came. Yes, I find myself on the wrong side of the exit door from the kinds of roles, responsibilities, and activities most people in our society consider significant. Yes, I find I can't quite get about as I used to. But the call is still there, calling even now, calling me to be what I am, and to discover now what it means to walk the way of aging. So there is an exciting future—*now*. And there's cause for curiosity for there may be surprises in store. And there's plenty of reason to keep alert and on my toes, for I have challenges to face. So realistic acceptance in faith can enkindle a creativity in an aging person that burns deep enough to survive being "left out" of the rush of younger society, and strong enough to keep him active in spite of the inertia that tends to set in when external demands decrease.

Involvement

Needless to say, this kind of acceptance is a far cry from taking all the frustrations of aging lying down. It is not resignation of the sort that leaves a person spiritless; it can fill a person with spark and vitality.

But it seldom does so directly in so many words. Like most things that occur at a certain spiritual depth, acceptance is most often unstated, expressed indirectly in the humor, strength, and style with which a person goes about his daily business. And so this basic attitude might reveal itself in some rather practical attitudes which are themselves based in profound acceptance.

One is an ability to keep interested in things. But this ability is most often the harvest of years of cultivation. Here an older person might advise the younger man to have a variety of interests besides his work, or might counsel the mother of growing children to develop skills and outlets for involvement that will provide fruitful channels and challenges for creative activity in later years. The temptation to devote all one's energy to work, or to dissipate all one's leisure time in passive occupations (such as constantly watching television), is from the perspective of the aging a deadly trap indeed. And the person who is realistic about himself will be wary of the things which tend to dim the spark of active curiosity and readiness for challenge within him.

Very important is the ability to share relationships with other people, the quality of availability that we have encountered earlier. Availability means the capacity to let go for a moment of one's self and one's own perspective, and enter the world and perspective of another person. And it means the capacity to share one's own world with that other person, to allow him inside. Such a relationship is a challenge in any case, but for the older person, especially if the person he encounters is considerably younger, the challenge is magnified.

Some problems of attitude need to be overcome if the aging person is to share significant relationships with others, at least others younger than he. First, the prejudice and stereotyping of the old that infects our culture may make a younger person reluctant to enter the world of his aging brother. On the other hand, the insecurity that the aging person may feel can cause him to close himself to others and compound his own sense of loneliness and abandonment.

If the older person tries to be conscious of the world of his younger companion, he can go a long way toward overcoming the barrier of prejudice. The younger man is in a world which the future dominates, and he tends to think of himself in terms of his hopes and plans rather than in terms of an unpretentious present. One so living toward the future is not likely to be more than mildly interested in the past, and so we shouldn't be terribly surprised if our "I remember when" stories draw a yawn. And a young man whose identity is caught up in plans and hopes is not likely to be receptive to the older and wiser man's realization that hopes fade and plans tend to go unfinished, for such a thought threatens him in a very radical way. Sensitivity and gentleness in the older person here may overcome a reluctance that too often prevents communication.

But there is a fear to open oneself to a younger person, based partially in the fear that he will not accept or respect what the aging person is and what he holds dear. "Old-fashioned ideas" are automatically bad, after all—or at least an aging person may feel that all younger people think so. But the fears that hinder availability can be overcome in two ways. First, by the strength and creativity that can be found through a realistic acceptance of himself, the aging person can quite confidently take the risk that he might be rejected as a "fuddy duddy." So what if he is? That's no reason he shouldn't try. Second, conversation can be directed or interpreted in ways that bring people together or that hold them apart. If the conversation, for instance, remains on the level of "shop-talk" and whatever happens to be on the surface of one's mind, then a workingman and a retired person are likely to find little in common, and a young mother and a widow may find that talking together takes some effort and some awkwardness. But if a person opens himself to another enough that common human concerns that lie beneath the surface of the mind are shared, then two persons of however different situations may discover an unsuspected richness in each other.

Of course, it is possible that they will find themselves in serious disagreement at that depth! Deeply held convictions about religion and morals and general philosophy of life may be utterly opposed, and some well-intentioned encounters can erupt into bitter conflict. Again availability is of the greatest importance. For one's convictions tend to arise out of the world of his experience, background, inner struggles, and commitments; they really make sense only in terms of that background. If we keep that in mind, we might have a chance at *understanding* someone who disagrees with us. An older man and his college-student nephew got into a furious argument about changes in Catholic attitudes toward morality. But each *listened* to each other and tried to understand what motives and reasons led him to think as he did. They have since remained close friends, for through their disagreement they came to understand each other as human beings.

(Incidentally, each has staunchly maintained his own opinion in regard to changes in Catholic attitudes toward morality.)

It is easier, of course, for relationships to develop between people who are in similar circumstances. And so an aging person is most likely to develop his significant relationships with those close to him in age. For that reason retirement communities have grown more and more popular, and through clubs and other social gatherings friendships among people going the same way are fostered. And that is good. After all, the difference between loneliness and friendship is just one other person.

Contributing

If we were to take literally many of the inspiring and optimistic things said and written about old age, then an aging person must be filled with wisdom and insight—treasures to pass on to his fellowman. But what he is more likely to feel is an uneasy sense of ambiguity, of *not* having all the answers, of failing to understand fully the world he lives in. And his uneasiness is the more disturbing because he no longer has the illusion of a glowing future when dreams come true. He knows that the ambiguity never goes away, and that dreams tend to become disappointment, while the temporary practical arrangements people make while they pursue their distant goals tend to become virtually permanent.

But perhaps there is a wisdom in that.

Reminder of the reality

In a culture caught up in a dream, a frenetic pursuit of an earthly paradise that isn't there, a desperately needed contribution is an occasional reminder of reality. Of course, genuine reminders of reality tend to be ignored or hidden by those who are caught up in the dream—but their presence is noted nonetheless, and their witness is significant. Disturbing as it may be to hear, there is a salutary value in the word spoken from one who stands near the end of the rainbow testifying that there waits no pot of gold.

And there is a contribution to be made in the very sense of ambiguity that is confirmed in the experience of the aging. For a person who has discovered the hollowness of dreams and promises is likely to be circumspect, slow to bite, when easy answers are offered. Wide experience and living through disappointment and disillusionment can equip a person with a 99%-effective delusion-detector. Time has provided him with a detailed tour of the junkyard where rust a thousand grand ideals and a thousand schemes to save the world, to build the earthly paradise. The way of aging knows better.

On the other hand, in the long perspective certain subtle and often overlooked values rise into relief, manifesting their goodness by their constancy. One ambitious professional man had pursued a lifetime career goal that seemed to evaporate as he grew older. Then he realized that the individual services he had performed, the individual persons he had aided, were his career goal. Another put it, "I sought to do my work in spite of interruptions, and distractions. Then I discovered that the interruptions *were* my work!" The person who seeks his meaning and value in his projects and ambitions can learn a valuable lesson from one who has discovered that meaning and value in the little things, the steps along the way. And the person who loses his self-respect because of failure in projects and ambitions can find reassurance.

In the process, though, of questioning the dreams and discovering some realities, a person in the way of aging can provide a significant alternative to the pursuit of paradise, a sense of values that is based in the present rather than the future, in the particular person, thing, or deed that faces him rather than the vague ideal, in what he is rather than in what he thinks he can make of himself.

Leisure

It is significant that for so many aging persons dreams of leisure give way to the disappointing reality of "nothing to do," a lack of significant activity. The aging person finds himself short-changed, and retirement brings less leisure than forced idleness. It is significant, for it is a symptomatic pain

revealing a disease or a lack in our culture—and unfortunately, it is a pain only subtly felt by those whose career are
still in full swing, but acutely felt by the aging. The aging
person then faces a challenge that is of real significance to his
fellowmen. By his calling attention to the pain, he gives notice
that something is wrong. And he can become a sort of pioneer
by seeking and perhaps discovering what it is whose absence
brings forth the pain.

It is a curious thing that the dictionary definition of
"leisure" makes the word roughly synonymous with "idleness." And "idleness" means not working. If we ponder the
fact that work is given extremely high value in our society and
is in fact how a man usually defines his identity, leisure
presents a real problem. Either leisure is understood in
relation to a person's work (I relax on the weekends so I can
come back to work Monday with a clear head), or it is a
totally unproductive and therefore meaningless situation.
This is a side effect of the "work ethic" that is so much of our
cultural heritage and that makes us a productive and progressive people. What the aging discover is that the "work
ethic" abandons its people in the end to lives that—because
they are "unproductive" in economic terms—are for all
practical purposes meaningless. What is lacking to the "work
ethic" and the society it dominates is precisely a true sense of
leisure.

But what is leisure, this holy grail that the aging seem
specially called upon to seek out?

Leisure fits into a way of thinking and a way of being that is
quite radically different from the "work ethic." In that way of
thinking, a person finds his identity and his meaning less in
what he does (though that is not unimportant) than in what
he *is*. And what he *is* is not so much a productive unit in an
economy as a conscious being who participates in a universe
that is itself filled with beauty and meaning. In his consciousness of himself and his world, the man of leisure seeks not
how to exploit his world or how to plan his career in it, but
seeks first of all to recognize and to rejoice in its beauty and

meaning. Utilitarian thoughts, economic concerns, are secondary to him; his mind rather tends toward the artistic, the poetic, ultimately the religious. For the meaning of the world reveals itself to him as *given* from a Being beyond, as reflecting the creative love of God. His response to its beauty, then, is more than pleasure at a pretty sight; it can be indeed a wordless prayer of praise and thanksgiving. Leisure is therefore an *attitude* rather than the condition of having time on one's hands. Ironically, the man of leisure can work quite effectively, whereas the man dominated by the "work ethic" discovers that leisure is a blind spot to him. He does not know how to relax in his being and appreciate the simple beauty of his world.

It is not surprising then that a person going through the magic door that leads out of a life of work discovers that it leads into a void. In a society which seems unable to fathom the meaning of a monk's or cloistered nun's life of contemplation and which perverts even a college education into vocational training, what else should he expect? There is no way provided for him—he must make his own way to a sense of leisure, or else suffer a kind of meaninglessness.

Of course, one solution that social theorists offer is to find fitting and productive employment for the aging: volunteer work, marketable handicrafts, etc. Such activities may help to deaden the pain the aging person feels in his "uselessness," and so it is a good thing. But the disease or lack in our culture remains.

Where is one to seek the holy grail of leisure? We can take a hint from the Grail Legend itself, and realize (as Percival learned) that the quest of the Grail is a spiritual quest. It may well begin with acceptance and its fruits—the relief that comes from not having to worry over a career ideal, the sense of affirmation and curiosity, the growing sensitivity to and appreciation for simple things, simply human things. From there it can go in countless directions.

At the wooded shore of a small and tranquil lake nestled in the Adirondack mountains, as the early morning mist rose from the smooth water to veil the mountain that towered beyond the lake, I met an old man sitting on a canvas camp stool and quietly sketching the beauty that he saw. With a silent sweep of his hand he directed my attention to the scene.

He didn't claim to be an artist, though he would spend a week or more pondering the morning lake and working most of the day with oil and canvas to produce a reasonably decent painting. What became of the paintings didn't concern him— he simply enjoyed the attempt to express the beauty that he recognized. Now, if this man had to feel useful in order to have a sense of being worthwhile, he would long before have become frustrated or bored with his painting. But he had learned to escape the world of work. The shades of light told him time, for the tyrant of the "work ethic," the clock, no longer had any hold on him. He kept his material needs simple, for he had come to delight simply in being.

He left that campground the morning after some self-conscious vacationers arrived with all the paraphernalia of what advertisers call "leisure"—including the inevitable loud radio (playing, of all things, news from New York City).

But the effect that this teacher of leisure had on me is such that very often unbidden there rises in my mind the clear image of smooth water breathing forth a mist to veil the mountain, and the silhouette of a man sitting still, gazing in contemplation.

Chapter 10

The Handicapped:
A Sign of Contradiction

From time to time an article appears in *The Reader's Digest* telling the triumphant story of a handicapped person who made it. Perhaps it is a youth who suffered from polio, but rose by sheer determination to become a great athlete and a prominent citizen. Perhaps it is a blind person who manages to run a successful business, or a paraplegic who manages to produce notable literary works.

Stories of this kind fill me with a sense of satisfaction the way a Walt Disney movie with a happy ending tends to do. But they raise some questions as well, questions that suggest unspoken attitudes or assumptions about the handicapped person. First, the general content of such stories follows a predictable pattern: how so-and-so overcame his handicap to achieve something that is admirable in the eyes of normal people, or how so-and-so won the respect of the normal world in spite of his handicap. There seems to be a suggestion then that the handicapped person has to compete with normal people and win in order to be respectable. Another question arises if I ponder the axiom that common occurrences never make news; only the exceptional story is news. Then such success for a handicapped person is exceptional, and failure— or being denied respect by the normal world—is the more common occurrence.

Despite the success stories, hero stories, and examples of what is possible for the handicapped person, the more common story is one of struggle, repeated frustration, and shattered self-respect. It is that story which calls for reflection here.

For the person with serious visual or hearing impairment, or for one who has lost the use of his limbs or through a nervous disorder cannot control his body as most people do, the struggle for some value and meaning in life is too often a long and painful one. Rehabilitation—the effort to develop what capacities a person has so that he can have a certain measure of independence and may even be able to support himself economically—is only the first step. More subtle and more complex than his physical disability is the disabling prejudice of the society he lives in, a society made up of people who consider themselves normal and who consider him different. The handicapped person is challenged to accept himself in spite of that prejudice, and then challenged further to live and act in a world that can be quite unsympathetic and cruel. But in this struggle, and in the common pain more truly than in the uncommon success, he stands as a sobering question raised to a society hypnotized by the pursuit of paradise.

Rehabilitation

The handicapped person discovers at nearly every turn that the world he lives in is built and managed by and for people with abilities he does not happen to have. Nevertheless, he is expected to fit into that world if he is going to survive. Perhaps "rehabilitation" can be described as the effort to fit a handicapped person as well as possible into the world of normal people.

The most immediate and acute problem the handicapped person faces is likely to be economic. To survive one must make a living, and to make a living one must work, and to work one must compete with normal people for jobs that require the skills and abilities of normal people. And so the most obvious goal of a rehabilitation effort will be to enable a handicapped person to make a living by some kind of economically productive work. Beneath the sheer economic need to work, however, there lurks a more subtle but deeper need. In a society that lives according to a "work ethic" and in which a person identifies himself by the kind of work he does, a man needs some kind of work in order to have a sense of self-respect, to claim a place among his fellowman as an equal.

But the goal of becoming employable is for many handicapped persons a distant one, and for many it is impossible. A nearer goal available to nearly everyone and achieved bit by bit is simply to gain some degree of independence. The ability to get around or at least some capacity for purposeful activity will mean escape from helplessness and so may mean a sense of worth to a person. A young victim of cerebral palsy, for instance, may take weeks to learn how to sit up unassisted. While his condition would seem pitable compared to the normal, this small achievement is significant for him as he is, and it marks a step along the road to greater and greater control of his body, and to an increased ability to care for himself even if he may never be fully employable. It is very unfortunate when efforts at rehabilitation are restricted to those who may become employable, for many of the severely handicapped may be deprived of any opportunity for greater self-respect and for lessened dependence upon others for care. Failing to value the lesser goals of rehabilitation suggests an unfortunate restriction of human worth to economic productivity.

The flip side of rehabilitation, however, is the effort to make some adjustments in the world to enable the handicapped to fit into it more easily. In most cities, a person who needs a wheelchair cannot avail himself of public transportation because access to it is barred to him by stairs or narrow doorways as effectively as a medieval castle was protected by a moat. How many buildings have set of steps before them which is impressive to the normal but impossible to one who cannot walk? Tragically, many people who depend on wheelchairs cannot even get in and out of their own homes without assistance, for most homes are designed for the normal even though the handicapped person is a member of a rather sizable minority.

There are many persons who are willing and able to work, but who require modified working conditions or special provisions because of their handicap. They cannot compete directly in the world of business and industry. Some provision is made for these by sheltered workshops designed specifically to provide employment for the severely handicapped. Such a program can make the difference between helplessness and some satisfying productive activity for the severely handicapped person. But there has been an unfortunate tendency for its contribution to the lives of the handicapped to remain rather limited. It is as if they should be satisfied to be able to do anything at all; and their rights and desires in relation to normal workers may be overlooked. After all, even severely handicapped persons would enjoy good tools and working conditions, an income that is adequate to support them, and some opportunity for advancement—things the normal worker is likely to demand. And so the very programs that lift a severely handicapped person from despair to some kind of hope may then unwittingly smother the hope that they have enkindled.

But the most prevalent problem that the rehabilitated handicapped person must face greets him when he tries to enter the world of normal people. Despite outstanding qualifications, despite the greatest effort and the strongest desire, he is likely to have a very difficult time finding employment that is adequate for him. Why? There are a number of words for it, such as "prejudice" or "discrimination," but the reality is tougher than any word can sound. When the handicapped person walks into the world of normal people, he is very likely to find denied him what is given without question to most of his fellowmen: acceptance as a human being.

The Big Problem

A young war veteran named Michael Jones returned to civilian life with a hook to replace the hand a shell had shattered. Months of work had made him proficient with the hook, so that he could perform nearly all manual tasks a normal person could. But he soon discovered that the physical disability of a handicap is only a small part of the reality of being a handicapped person. The big problem is being visibly *different*. He got into the habit of subtly concealing his differentness as well as he could. And so he might enter a conversation in a store or at a party, only to see his companion's face suddenly freeze when the hook was revealed, and the conversation would become hopelessly awkward. He found it impossible to get a date with a girl who had seen him as he was. He found that for all practical purposes his entire personality in all its complexity and with all of its strengths was reduced to one metal hook, and that was the only thing people noticed about him.

A handicap that makes a person visibly different from the normal person does tend to force itself on attention, with the result that what someone is likely to see in him is not the person but simply the handicap. And so instead of sharing an emotionally neutral meeting of persons, the handicapped person finds himself faced with a confused and awkward reaction to the visible handicap—an attitude of disgust and rejection or of pitying protectiveness. He is not generally given the chance to be known as the full person that he is.

The handicap then becomes the one trait by which the person is recognized and identified. This veteran's name may be Sergeant Mike Jones, but his name might as well be Captain Hook.

Mike's identity may be undercut further as generalizations are made about him on the basis of his visible differentness. First, he is regarded as "handicapped." Unfortunately, that is a rather broad category which includes the deaf, the blind, all amputees, the hopelessly palsied, and the severely retarded, among others. Such is the nature of a stereotype, however, that all handicapped persons are regarded as "helpless cripples," and often tactlessly treated as such. Further, his handicap, limited as it is, is regarded as the model for his whole personality. Hence he is expected to be handicapped in practically every way, and he is surprised to find people trying to help him sit down, or holding doors for him. This problem is especially present with a disability which touches a primary sense of a person. So for instance a blind person may find to his irritation that a well-meaning helper begins to support him as if he were crippled, or to speak very loud as if he were hard of hearing. Finally, since the handicapped is considered so generally disabled, anything normal he does is a surprise to his companions. Were Mike to stand and run, he might astonish those who regard him basically as an attachment to his hook. For a blind man to light a cigarette without faltering may cause gasps of amazement. In each case, the handicapped person is perceived as a handicap, and not really as the person that he is.

Most painful, though, is that his differentness is understood—sometimes in so many words, sometimes unconsciously—as inferiority.

Especially if his ability to work is affected by his handicap, a person is likely to be looked down upon. Once again the world of the "work ethic" hits a limit, for within it personal worth is evaluated in terms of achievement—education, function in society, productivity, money. A person who is not fully productive is often considered a burden to society. "What good is he?" The tendency to measure a man's worth in terms of his productive capacity is most cruelly exemplified in discussions regarding the abortion of a fetus likely to have a deformity. High-sounding concerns for "quality of life" or a "life that is worthwhile" may have beneath them an unstated but clearly present assumption that the capacity to participate in the productive endeavors of normal people is essential for human worth and human happiness. The unemployable handicapped person is told in effect, especially if his defect is congenital, that it would be better had he never been born. What effect would such a thought have on a person's self-respect?

The very *differentness* of a person can become not only a distraction from his other personal qualities, but a detraction from his very worth as a person. The most obvious instances of cruel intolerance for differentness are found among children, where a quality that sets a child apart from the rest of the group makes him the target of taunts and jeers, and often results from his exclusion from the group. Perhaps from a kind of herd instinct, a sense of insecurity in oneself that causes a person to identify with a group and look down on those who are "out" is at the root of such intolerance. Whatever its root, its butt is likely to be the handicapped person. Young children stare at him, strangers approach with pitying words though no one invited their concern, potential employers wrinkle brows, and those he might desire to love turn from him.

Apparently people just don't like to have a handicapped person around. There is something disturbing to the normal person about the presence of an obvious handicap. The effortful movements of a palsied person cause the normal person to turn from his path so as not to meet him. The unseeing gaze of a blind man in a restaurant causes some customers to feel queasy. So the pursuit of paradise that gave us the get-well card appears to have equipped us with a revulsion against reminders of the vulnerability and limits of our nature. The presence of the handicapped in our world shouts too loudly of its imperfection: we cannot bear to have them. And so the handicapped find themselves, like the sick and the aging, advised to hide themselves from the normal people, the chasers of rainbows, or at least to have the good manners to keep their ugliness as unobtrusive as possible.

Coping

Despite the occasional success stories, the lot of the handicapped person is generally tough. He faces a challenge in coming to know, accept, and affirm himself as the person he is. He faces a further challenge in dealing with the people he encounters, people who respond to him not as the person he is but as a grotesque. And he finds on top of all that a call addressed to him to make a specific contribution to a society which needs him to remind it of reality.

Accepting himself

The person with a visible handicap suspects that he may be a person. He knows the range of powers, the depth of feeling, the breadth of awareness, and the personal history that makes him what he is. Like every other human being, he senses that he is good (while he may secretly fear he is not), and he wants others to regard him and accept him in the richness of his whole personality.

And yet he cannot avoid being aware that he is different. The community in which he lives reflects to him an attitude of curiosity, awkwardness or even rejection—setting him apart. His own family of upbringing may have communicated to him some of the dismay, pity, or overprotectiveness that suggests that he is not really a person quite like others. And as a result he himself may have a deep sense of inferiority and even of worthlessness. The kind of inner strength and determination that makes for the success story is undermined in him perhaps from birth.

As he recognizes that he is not like other people, there is apparently something "wrong" with him that he can do nothing about, he may feel a kind of rebellion within him. But since rebellion against a sheer fact is rather fruitless, the rebellion may settle into a simmering bitterness that can have poisonous effects. *Why me?* Again it is the question of Job— and again there is no direct answer to it.

There is no *why*, there is only the real situation. But in that situation it is possible to recognize not an unjust affliction but a call—a simple call to *be* what you are, even if that cannot be measured by the standards of value shared by most people. There is no profound philosophy in responding to that call, for it is as simple as an unspoken will to go on living. But in its simplicity, the will to go on living without bitterness can have profound roots. A person can recognize in his handicap the call of one who gives a value to him that is beyond question, beyond rejection. He knows he is worthwhile, no matter what others think of him. And he knows he is worthwhile precisely as he is—the whole person that he is *including* his handicap, not "in spite of" his handicap.

Ironically, it is this very acceptance of himself as he is that can be the ground of another kind of rebellion. For self-acceptance does not mean that a handicapped person feels the obligation of fitting into the stereotype of "helpless cripple" that the society of normal people may apply to him. It means affirming what one is, even asserting what one is and can become. A sense of worth in oneself that is grounded in firm faith can then become a standpoint in a kind of conflict.

The conflict is immediately apparent to him as soon as he affirms within himself the person that he is. For this self-affirmation gives him the expectation that others will regard him as he regards himself, while experience will lead him to expect others to regard him simply in terms of his handicap. He knows he is not likely to get a "fair hearing" before the unspoken judgment of those with whom he deals.

When he is among normal people, he will still feel a kind of self-consciousness, almost a nakedness. The human failings of his companions are clothed with the protection of privacy— but the man with a visible handicap has his short-comings displayed before anyone who chooses to look. He cannot participate in the charade of flawless respectability—his companions exhibit the kind of polite awkwardness toward him that they might show toward a prominent person whose arrest for drunken driving has just appeared in the morning paper. Beneath the small talk and behind the curious glances there is an unspoken major topic of conversation, and the handicapped person has a rather clear idea of what kind of things will be said as soon as he leaves the group.

In spite of himself he feels a shame for his handicap. And so he finds within himself a disturbing conflict between the worthwhile self he affirms and the shameful oddity he is made to feel he is to others. Almost angry with himself, he realizes that he is judging himself according to the notion of "normal" that his companions assume, and so of course coming up short. This inner conflict, however, may bring him to realize something significant. What is truly "normal?" Is it an abstract and idealized image of a "whole man" that is imposed on everyone, and in relation to which *everyone* falls short— though some more visibly than others? If so, then the "normal" companions who consider him an oddity are arrogant indeed, as if they measured up and he didn't. But in fact there is no abstract and idealized image that can be imposed. The normal situation among human beings is *diversity*: a wide range of different possibilities describe what a human being should be. And the handicapped person fits within that notion of "normal." The true normal, he may realize, is not a leveling common mold, but a richness and variety that makes human society the intricate tapestry that it is. Through his inner conflict, therefore, provided he is grounded in a firm self-affirmation, the handicapped person can come to the simple recognition that his "normal" companions are just plain *wrong*. They are blind to the human reality, and they have a crippled consciousness, while being completely unaware of the assumptions which so blind and cripple them.

But that realization does not change anything in the situation of a handicapped person. Now he has a double handicap: his physical disability and a clear misunderstanding that results in a kind of social disability. Can he accept not only his own handicap but the handicap of the society he lives in?

He has several options in his attitude toward "normal" society. If his handicap sets him significantly apart (as total blindness might), he may choose to associate primarily with others who share his handicap, and so live for the most part in a segregated world where his handicap is not a block to acceptance. He may choose to attempt living in the "normal" world by learning to function in a way as close to normal as possible. Or he may exploit his given role as an oddity, and find his place in normal society by acting out the stereotype of the "helpless cripple." Tragically, none of these options allows him really to be himself. The tension or conflict between what he knows himself to be and what his social situation expects him to be challenges him to achieve a delicate balance if he is to be true to himself and still get along. Ironically, he is called to develop a sensitivity, tact, and self-reliance that is actually far in excess of that demanded of the "normal" person. (How sweet it is to have such a high vocation! he might say sarcastically). And yet that is his challenge.

Getting along in polite society

Perhaps simply because he is a human being, a handicapped person wants to share in the life of normal society. Depending on just how visible his handicap is, and how decisively it draws the attention of those whom he encounters, the problem he faces will vary. Perhaps he will be able to pass for just another person, and so achieve the distinction among the handicapped of arousing no particular notice. He may find his handicap impossible to hide, and so he is challenged to make the best of the awkwardness felt in his encounters. In any case, he is likely to find that there are limits to his acceptance by polite society, and like the black man encountering the white liberal suburbanite he has to know his place. The world of the get-well card touches him quite clearly.

For some, a handicap can be corrected or compensated for well enough so that the person does not appear in any way different from the normal. An amputee may be fitted with an artificial leg and become so proficient in walking with it that "only his doctor knows." A young woman with severe myopia can be fitted with contact lenses that adequately correct her vision and allow her to dispense with the thick glasses that she feels would make her ugly. A totally deaf person may be so adept at lip reading and reading others' reactions that his handicap may go unnoticed in most conversations.

For these, there is little problem entering polite society on an equal footing with the normal person. The problem is felt in his fear of being discovered. The young woman is careful never to be seen wearing her thick glasses. The amputee wonders what he would do if he spilled hot coffee on his artificial limb—and failed to react. The deaf person is careful to avoid situations where he cannot be facing his companion without awkwardness.

The effort to pass for normal can mean a real tension and anxiety for the handicapped person, especially if he has not fully and objectively accepted himself as he is. Sometimes the tension can lead him to make decisions that are contrary to his best interest: If Mike Jones, for instance, wanted more than anything to appear normal, he might avail himself of an artificial hand which looks normal (at least from a distance) but is not functional. For the sake of appearance, he might deprive himself of the real ability that a hook would provide for him. A minor but very common example of this tendency is the habit of many people with relatively minor visual impairment to go without glasses in public, even though they may not be able to see quite clearly or read without eyestrain. The more desperate the desire to pass for normal and the fear of being exposed in one's handicap, the more likely a person is to fall for faddish and overpriced miracle cures or compensating gimmicks—the handicapped person sets himself up for victimization.

But if he accepts himself, his effort to pass for normal loses its desperate quality. He attempts to appear as normal as possible almost as a service to his companions. If he "blows his cover," he will be able frankly to laugh about his situation, and patiently to endure the inevitable prying questions about how he lost his leg or how he can manage so well with such a handicap. As he goes on with that group of companions, of course, he will never again be taken for "normal," but rather will be accorded the anomalous distinction as a handicapped person that you really wouldn't know was handicapped. Within himself, he needs a deeper sense of humor to accept a world in which he cannot frankly be himself, but must rather play games to get along: games at which he may be quite adept, but games nonetheless.

The person who cannot hide his handicap has another kind of game to learn, the ability to offset or overcome the uneasiness or awkwardness that his condition imposes on his encounters.

He himself can never be sure just how a stranger will react to him, and so he may with good reason dread every new encounter. He may be utterly rejected—being politely ignored is the form that takes in polite society. Or on the other extreme he may be subjected to gushing and patronizing imposition: "Oh, you poor thing, how you must suffer, please *do* let me help you." In between he will encounter in various disguises a tendency to focus attention on the one quality to which he is reduced, his handicap. Seldom does he encounter a person who greets him simply as a human being, and pays the kind of attention to his handicap that might be paid to something like hair color in a normal person.

Patience is likely to be needed as a basic tactic. The do-gooder who rushes in to help him do things he is perfectly capable of managing himself might deserve a deftly disguised admonition to mind his own business. But ironically the handicapped person is called upon to take into account the awkwardness this person feels, and accept their misguided but well-intentioned offers for the sake of placing them at ease. The disguised curiosity of others may have to be met squarely and settled, even if that means the handicapped person's sufferings become a public matter. The pain of being ignored may simply have to be endured. But there the patience of the handicapped can be stretched to its limit: a blind man in a large city found it nearly impossible to stop a passerby in order to find out at what intersection he stood. "Excuse me, could you . . ." and the approaching steps would continue on by or turn away.

But his strategy will be to do everything he can to make it easier for those he meets to withdraw their attention from his handicap and turn it to the kind of common meeting ground that topics of conversation usually provide in polite society. He will try to act as much at ease as possible with himself, and interact with others in ways which will not be distracting. A blind man, for instance, may find it helpful to turn his face toward the person to whom he speaks, even though it is a sightless gaze that he directs. If he does not, the sighted person to whom he speaks is distracted by the discrepancy from the usual pattern of communication, and may get the feeling that real communication is not taking place.

The handicapped needs to be skilled at his game, for the normal person is not likely to be able to adapt to him. And so the handicapped needs to know how to make the first move in a conversation, how to confront and overcome the awkwardness that the other person feels. After all, he has to play that game in his every encounter, so he has the opportunity to become quite practiced at it. And so he is given a further responsibility. Not only must he physically adapt to his handicap and cope with the stigma placed on him by a society which fails to understand, he must also take the responsibility of helping the members of that society deal with his handicap in spite of their own blindness to human reality and crippled consciousness.

The handicapped person is called upon, in short, to have a heroic inner strength and generosity.

The temptation is attractive to withdraw into the closed society of those who share his handicap and to make no big deal of it. But another temptation that can be seriously counter-productive is present, too. The handicapped person may become alarmed at the uneasiness of others in dealing with him, the more disturbed by it the more he feels he needs approval and support from others. He is threatened by a kind of panic. He may try to demand of others an understanding that they don't have, or if he finds a glimmer of understanding he may want to cling to that person, seeking emotional support and constant reinforcement and even help. That will of course tend to drive the other from him, and the normal people with whom he deals may tend more and more to avoid him simply out of fear of the demands he will place on them. A downward spiral thus begins which leaves the handicapped person ever more desperate, and the people around him ever more reluctant to deal with him until he is threatened by a serious emotional crisis.

Acceptance and patience—coupled with a sense of humor—may be a difficult and challenging way, but that is about the only way that can be fruitful.

The fruit it bears, though, is limited, and in the end the handicapped person is likely to learn that no real option open to him allows him really to be himself. For the handicapped person who has managed to get along in polite society needs to stay within certain limits. A double amputee, for instance, may have gained some acceptance from a circle of normal friends as he sits in his wheelchair. But in his own private home he gets around passably by dragging himself along with his arms. Let him try that among tolerant friends and there would be screams! The acceptance he is given by normal people may be sincere, but it extends only so far. The handicapped person is accepted, yes, and advised that he is just as good as normal folks. But he must know his place, and not make the demands on his normal friends that they take a good realistic look at him and accept him as he actually is.

Such is the challenge to get along in polite society.

Making A Contribution Anyway

If the handicapped person accepts his own limits and the limits of the human situation with a sense of humor and a faith that hopes for more than justice, the obvious injustices he faces need not result in bitterness. Bitterness at injustice, after all, grows from the same root as the get-well card: the expectation that there should be a kind of paradisal order on earth, and so an impatience with anything that is not as it should be. On the other hand, it need not result in a sort of hopeless resignation that delusions shall never be shattered or injustices never overcome. There are significant contributions the handicapped person is well placed to make to his fellowmen—contributions that may not be immediately appreciated, but perhaps the more significant for that. The first kind of contribution he makes simply by his ability to function as a human being. The second he can make by dramatizing the anomaly of his position in society.

A quiet witness

It is a truism that we are all handicapped in some way or another. A man of fifty is not expected to play professional football, nor is a child expected to carry out a task that requires months or years of work. The implication of the truism is that there should be no particular shame in being handicapped in a less common way. But the truth of the matter is that there is shame in being handicapped—yet we are all handicapped in one way or another. It is just that my handicap is a secret moral or psychological failing that only I know or only my intimates guess. And the analogy would be complete if my hidden faults would be made as plain to see as the white cane of the blind man or the limp of the partially paralyzed. I know the embarrassment I would feel—and so I can only wonder at the calm nonchalance that the handicapped may have achieved.

There is a hidden sadness that most people feel—a sense of not being what we could or should be, perhaps of being quite unworthy of another's respect or regard. Some feel it as a pain and tend to withdraw, some compensate for it by an aggressive assertion and come on strong. But beneath the respectable mask that every person more or less unconsciously wears to get along in polite society, there is likely to be a sense of phoniness or hypocrisy, precisely in being accorded the kind of acceptance that is given to the "normal" individual, the unblemished specimen of humanity.

In a way, the obviously handicapped person has the advantage of having his claim to undeserved respect undercut by a visible failing, preventing him from collaborating in what might be thought of as a rather general hypocrisy. And at the very least, the handicapped person who maintains a positive attitude toward himself and who continues to live as full a human life as is possible for him can become a kind of sign. In the dark times, seeing a discrepancy between what we know we are and what others think of us, in the times when we have a difficult time accepting ourselves for partial beings rather than paragons, the steady effort to cope made by the palsied or the blind can be like a beacon to a lost ship. There is a place for us, and a value for us, handicapped though we be.

A salutary scream of anger

But chances are, the generality of normal folk prefer to be left in their complacency, and allowed to maintain the charade of respectability as unblemished specimens of humanity. That may explain why the presence of the handicapped tends to be rather carefully veiled for most people.

The unpleasant fact is that the handicapped person finds himself faced with a conflict of values—what he knows he is, and what society generally expects him to be. His needs and even demands tend to be met by half-measures, very much like the gushy helpfulness of the person who gives demonstrative but irrelevant help for a moment, but is unlikely to stay around long enough to learn what help the handicapped person really could use. It takes little subtlety to see that the purpose of giving such help is less to meet the need of the handicapped than to assuage the "social conscience" of the helper.

The handicapped person finds that his efforts to cope by acceptance, patience, and concern for the comfort of the normal person has an unavoidable negative effect. If he does get along in polite society, he does so in a way which very effectively prevents his normal companions from having to face their own assumptions—assumptions that the handicapped knows are just plain *wrong*. He appears comfortable in his differentness in order to put his companions at ease. But they are thereby insulated from the pain of his situation. He adapts himself to a world that is ill fitted to his needs, and his normal companions marvel at his ingenuity and determination and forget that a few changes in laws regarding building design, accessibility to public transportation, etc., would enable him to adapt much more effectively without the tremendous waste of effort he now must make. He is careful to minimize his differentness—and thereby his normal companions are prevented from confronting the clear contradiction to the earthly paradise that he presents.

There is frustration in having to play games in order to get along in polite society, for one cannot simply relax and be himself. But there is a strategic advantage to that, too. For if the handicapped person knows he is playing a game, and more or less consciously protecting his normal friends from his handicap, then it is in his power to shift at a strategic moment to being dead serious, and reveal the unresolved conflict that is buried beneath polite tolerance. The handicapped person is treated "just like one of us"—and it is in his power to demonstrate the ironic implication of that cliche. He can unmask the blindness to true humanity and the crippled consciousness that is part of the cultural disease we have called the pursuit of paradise.

But his scream of anger, justified in itself as a reaction to the prejudice that complicates his life even more than his physical handicap does, can mean for the society he lives in a call to a greater humanity.

For he is calling on his fellow men to scrap the illusory idea of "normality" as an ideal type and replace it with an awareness of the variety and complexity that fits within the range of "normal" human life-styles. He is calling on them to abandon a standard of judging persons that demands a conformity to expectations and excludes those who are different, and replace it with a positive standard of evaluating that seeks the richness that each differing person has to offer. He is calling for a social world in which he will be recognized and judged for what he is in the fullness of his personality, rather than being reduced to the one perhaps minor aspect of his being that makes him visibly different from others.

He is calling for a change of heart, really—perhaps the most impossible but the most important demand that any person can make of a society.

But that is after all the very demand that is made by Christianity. And the call of Christianity is a call to share in Christ's overcoming the realm of death, where failures and inadequacies dominate, and bringing the realm of God, where justice and love are set free by a God who forgives and who loves enough not only to heal the blind, deaf, and lame, but to forgive the sinner.

Chapter 11

A Painful Truth In Mental Illness

As we reflect from a Christian perspective on a concept of health that includes sickness, certain kinds of mental illness take on a special significance. We have said that this ideal of health is wholeness and integrity, an image of life or a set of attitudes that gives place to every aspect of life, and makes of life a unified sense, a harmonious whole. But such health is an ideal rather than a state of mind the majority of people have without struggle. We have seen how many forces in our society encourage us to ignore what speaks of human limitations, and to pretend that an earthly paradise is almost in our grasp. But when a person comes to see through that dream and collides with the sometimes terrifying reality of his limits, the struggle he goes through can take the form of a mental illness.

The kinds of mental illness that are especially relevant here are those that arise through the anxiety and stress a person suffers as he tries to cope with himself and his situation. Some mental disorders have clearly physical causes: an injury to the brain, or a disease which affects the nervous system. But many arise as a desperate effort to cope with crises or failures or inadequacies—or simply with the terrifying finiteness of the human condition that is symbolized, for example, in those rather common dreams of threats to one's life. These mental illnesses portray a painful truth. And for the one who suffers them they can mean disintegration—coming apart at the seams—or the way to a new harmony, a scarred but profound integrity.

194

How Normal Is Normal?

Definitions of the "normal" personality are generally very tentative if they are given at all, for while certain types of abnormal behavior can be clearly described, normality is hard to pin down. Perhaps the simplest way to distinguish the normal person from the mentally ill is to realize that all persons have to cope with the real situation in which they live. The normal person develops habits, attitudes, and actions which enable him to live with a certain amount of comfort in his situation, and without too much anxiety or stress. He is therefore called a "well-adjusted" person. But if his habits, attitudes, and actions are not so successful, if they are inappropriate or cause anxiety or stress of increasing severity, the chances are his behavior will reflect one or another pattern characteristic of mental illness.

It should then be quite clear that there are *degrees* of normality and *degrees* of mental illness, and normality and mental illness shade into each other the way colors on a spectrum do: they are not two neatly separated ways of being. Normality and mental illness can be present in a person at once, for mental illness affects only certain aspects of a personality, leaving him perfectly normal in most of his personality. Further, if we understand a mental illness not as some wierd visitation on a person but simply his desperate but misguided effort to cope with his situation, then mental illness is a perfectly understandable part of life the way physical illness is. Since most people are not entirely successful in their efforts to cope with reality, most people are likely to be a mixture of the "well-adjusted" and the "inappropriate," and most people are likely to have a certain amount of anxiety and a reasonable ration of eccentricities.

The very fact that mental illness exists is a signal that coping with reality can be a difficult challenge, and true mental health—*integrity*, which may be something more than being "well-adjusted"—is not something to be taken for granted.

It is, in fact, possible to turn the picture of normality and mental illness upside down. There can be something unhealthy about a person who is perfectly well-adjusted to an awful situation—the extremely effective soldier in war, for example. Some situations *should* cause extreme stress and tension—and "adjustment" to them could indicate a complete lack of sensitivity in a person. A magazine cartoon showed a psychiatrist telling an obviously terrified patient in a padded cell, "you are the one who is sane; the others are crazy, but they are in charge."

There can be an unhealthy complacency in the "well-adjusted" person. After all, isn't it a bit ironic to point at a distressed person and say "he can't cope," when we who point live in a society which tends carefully to mask and hide from itself painful and threatening aspects of reality? Perhaps there is something basically questionable about a person who can feel completely at ease in a society which calmly sits on a stockpile of nuclear weapons adequate to propel the earth into another galaxy, or which argues and struggles and finally refuses to invest some millions in feeding a hungry world while billions are spent without blinking on more and deadlier military weapons. Is "adjustment" to such a situation healthy, even though that is the way currently to avoid anxiety and stress?

What we call "mental illness" then may need to be understood in a more positive light. Is it possible that among those who are comfortably "normal" are many who are simply *unaware* of the full dimensions of their situation? And is it possible that what we call "mental illness" comes as a result of a person's encounter with the full reality in which he lives—including the sinister and threatening tendencies that are part of himself and his world, and the dark limits that are simply a basic dimension of the human condition? Mental illness then may mean for the person who suffers it a call to a deeper health—to an integrity profound enough to take fully into account that dark side of reality.

Confronting The Dark Side

Mental illness might be thought of as part of a process of change in a person. It is less an unfortunate accident which happens to him, as an unconscious effort on his part to meet demands placed on him. These demands may be buried in his unconscious, or may be too deep for clear expression in the words and symbols of consciousness. Inappropriate as his habits, attitudes, or actions may seem, it is likely then that there is a sort of logic to his illness, "a method to his madness," when it is understood in terms of the demand it so desperately attempts to meet. The symptoms of abnormality may well arise then when a person recognizes a need to change the stance toward life that he has taken in the past, a stance that is inadequate. And they will be likely to disappear when he arrives at a new stance. When a person emerges from a mental illness, he may not be "the same as he always was," for he is likely to have a much more profound, more humble, and more realistic relationship to his world than he had in the past.

The sense of deep anxiety that is an aspect of many mental illnesses might be described as a strong but undefined fear for one's well being. It is a fear that is as gripping as that felt by a person whose automobile goes into a skid at high speed—only that person has the benefit of knowing precisely what it is that threatens him, whereas anxiety is a response to a threat which cannot be readily identified. If that person would develop a fear that made him very uneasy every time he entered an automobile, his fear would be on the way to becoming anxiety.

Anxiety comes in many colors, to match a variety of threats to one's well-being. All such threats are vague and have no specific object. If they had, the person could address himself specifically to that and deal directly with the cause of his fear once and for all. But they do not. For the most part, such anxiety arises in response to threats or limits that are part of the human condition. Mental illness is not just a matter of *sensing* these threats, for they are normal. It is a matter of failing to incorporate them effectively into himself.

The person who has been in dangerous skid may develop as a result a whole set of fears—heights, enclosed places, dark city streets, storms—that are rooted in his very direct experience of the possibility of sudden death. Can one say his fears are exaggerated? After all, sudden death is a very real possibility for any person at any time. Learning to live with the stark recognition of that possibility is not easy.

A common source of anxiety is a sense of being unacceptable or unlovable, a sense of inadequacy as a person. Such an anxiety can produce an unrealistic effort to be perfect and pleasing to everyone, combined with a hesitancy and lack of assertiveness that stems from being unsure of others' acceptance. All this is within the normal range of suffering unless it reaches an extreme form, a neurosis, that seriously interferes with a person's ability to function. The logic behind it might run this way: I am meaningless unless I am accepted and loved, and I have to deserve acceptance and love by being so good no one can object to me. One sad irony is that his efforts to be perfect and his transparent begging for acceptance tend to repel people from him, making him even more desperately redouble the obsequious efforts to be perfect. The other sad irony is that he knows deep down he is not perfect and so he feels unsure of whatever love he is given. He may "test" others' love for him, making himself a problem in the process. All this can occur within the normal range of human suffering—and it is a frequent theme in fiction and on TV serials. In its extremes it can become a neurosis—perhaps a painstaking perfectionism that paralyzes a person and makes it impossible for him ever to finish a task, or perhaps a kind of unreasoning jealousy that demands constant assurance of love and is nevertheless consistently suspicious of infidelity. The profound truth beneath such an anxiety is that all real love is really undeserved—it is a free gift, a grace. And the ultimate love which means salvation is something beyond earning, beyond achieving, and beyond any human adequacy. Beneath the anxiety then may be the realization that one's meaning and acceptability are completely beyond his control. And that can be a fearful thought.

Parallel to the anxiety which arises from having one's relationship with others beyond complete control is an anxiety from a world that seems chaotic, out of control, unpredictable—a world that includes one's own powers. Unable to live at ease in a world in which little remains stable, a person may desperately try to build around himself a perfectly ordered, safe world, where there is a place for everything and everything in its place. The most obvious manifestation of this tendency is the housewife whose home is always so clean and orderly that it makes any guests and even her family vaguely uncomfortable, or it may be manifest in a person who has a fanatical concern for law and order, in its extreme the person who sees plots and "international conspiracies" threatening everywhere. Here the neurosis is rapidly approaching a more serious condition called paranoia. Unable to live at ease with himself because of undesirable or wild tendencies he senses in himself a person who may maintain a rigorous personal discipline that would make a monastery seem lenient by comparison. The tension of keeping oneself under so tight a lid may manifest itself in many ways. Within the context of religion, a person may seek to purify himself of everything even slightly resembling a fault, and then grow more and more sensitive to the tiniest imperfections. Once such a tendency was praised as the development of a pure conscience, but since Jansenism has gone out of style and psychological insight has influenced our understanding of religious behavior, this tendency is recognized as scrupulosity, a form of obsessive-compulsive neurosis. Or the tension may find another expression in a reversal—a very disciplined person may suddenly burst out of his self-imposed prison and indulge the very tendencies he feared so much that they grew stronger and stronger within him. Again the mental illness is a very logical but inadequate response to a very real anxiety—

the anxiety that comes from having one's world and one's own life beyond control, out of one's own hands.

Perhaps the most stark manifestation of anxiety is the nameless, incomprehensible, overpowering dark force that is described by some who have suffered severe mental illness and come out of it scarred but whole. The efforts to give that anxiety a name and to manage it produce the milder problems we have glanced at. But when it presents itself without disguise, the simple and overpowering threat of absolute chaos, absolute meaninglessness and nothingness, there is no managing it. It is as if one falls into a vast dark chasm, an abyss. And so a person "snaps"—he flees in terror from what is unendurable but inescapable. Or else, convinced of the ultimate futility of his dreams and hopes, stung by failure, he may simply turn completely off, totally separate himself from all activity and effort and human contact. And who can say that his response is not perfectly logical in the face of the ultimate darkness that clouds the human condition?

It is a painful thing to confront the dark side of oneself and of the reality in which one lives—especially if up to that point a person has lived in the reassuring complacency of an easy "normality." It is as if the firm ground on which we walk so confidently were to dissolve, and we discover that we stand suspended over a dark abyss, delicately walking a tightrope and fearing to look down. When the surface of life dissolves, the reassuring routine of daily activities that gives us a sense of who we are and where we stand shatters with it, leaving us with the terrifying sense of threatening emptiness, and the temptation to despair of any meaning or worth in life at all. As one fights to keep his balance over that abyss, he may resort to behavior that seems odd to one who thinks he is standing on solid ground. And if one feels himself falling, there is no describing his terror.

One Way Through

There are a number of approaches to the treatment of mental illness. One school of psychology suggests that most disorders can be traced to a trauma or an emotional hunger that went unsatisfied in childhood, and so it will direct the person who seeks help to dig into his early years and revive his earliest memories. Another looks to the powers of the unconscious mind to probe, reveal, and even solve complex psychological problems, and counsels a person to examine his behavior in the light of dreams. Another seeks to help a person see himself objectively, and so the psychologist attempt to act as a mirror, reflecting a person's feelings and thoughts back to him so he can see them as they are. Some see the basic root of psychological problems in the person's attempt to keep the lid on his urges and instincts, especially his sexual drives. Some see it in the attempt to adjust successfully to his situation, especially his emotional situation. And others see it in the quest within a person for wholeness and meaning.

But a human being is complex, and human life has the marvelous character of living itself out on many levels at once, and in many dimensions at once. So it is that any one of a variety of approaches can be of help to a person struggling with mental illness, for growth in one dimension of life most often implies or even brings about growth in its other dimensions.

There is one dimension of the struggle for wholeness that is fundamental to life, but one most often not directly followed. Perhaps that is best. This dimension is the religious, that aspect of one's being in which he holds himself in relation to God, one way or another. And perhaps it is best that the way of religion is not often directly followed for it is too easy to turn religion into a set of cushions for complacency, a set of platitudes that hide the abyss and so prevent a person from confronting the painful truth, the dark side of human reality. But that does not mean that the profound reality of religion is not *there*, at work beneath and within the other dimensions of a person's struggle. And that does not mean that the solution a person comes to, the more profound, humble, and realistic relationship to his world that a mental illness may bring him to, is not fundamentally a religious realization whether or not it is recognized as such.

From the point of view of our Christian reflections on mental illness, it is important to look more closely at the religious dimension, the religious way through mental illness. That is not to suggest religion as a method of psycho-therapy—it most probably would not work. But it is to bring to light the Christian significance of mental illness, and perhaps to discover the meaning it has in relation to a Christian understanding of the world.

Some counsel acceptance

It is possible to look at the various forms of neurosis and even some more serious mental illnesses as desperate defenses a person unconsciously constructs to ward off from himself that fearsome dark side of himself or of reality. Over a number of years, the defenses may develop defenses of their own, so that a person's mental state is like a labyrinth of habits and attitudes that correspond to his inner fears and may be quite inappropriate in relation to his outer world. A psychologist may be able to help such a person find his way back through the labyrinth to the trauma, the unacceptable aspect of himself or of reality that promoted this uncon-sciously constructed fortress in the first place. A phrase used to describe this process is "peel the onion"—getting through layer after layer of defenses in order to discover and deal with the basic problem that the person has not been able to solve.

Once that problem is discovered and laid bare, the theory goes, its compelling power over the person is broken and he can accept himself once again. If he does so accept himself, then he will no longer need the layers of defenses that have built up—perhaps in the form of neurotic behavior—and they will disappear like fog before the warm rays of the sun. He will then be freed to act spontaneously and appropriately and generously in a relationship to himself and his world that is healthy and adequate.

But the way of acceptance is more complex than that.

If the dark side of oneself is unacceptable and repelling, it is so not just because it is buried in the unconscious. It *is* threatening, and to admit it is there can amount to a rather thorough demolition of one's self-image. And so systematically to lay bare the hidden horrors within a person is no guarantee that he will look on them and be able to laugh in realistic self-acceptance. If the dark side of reality is terrifying, it is not so just because it enters a person's mind in the form of grotesque images. It *is* terrifying, and to be brought face-to-face with it can amount to being marched before a firing squad without benefit of blindfold. And so systematically to confront a person with the abyss and then try to veil it by such platitudes as "everyone has to face it" is more like a feeble attempt to revive the complacency of the "normal" than a genuine resolution.

And yet such efforts to uncover and face such terrifying aspects of reality are very often successful, and the suffering person is often able to accept himself as he is, dark side and all, and to accept the human condition, complete with the abyss that lies beneath the surface of living.

Evidently there is more at work than simply uncovering the problem, for the effect is out of proportion to the cause.

How can a person be at ease with himself when he knows that within him lie forces that can undo every good thing he has lived for? How can a person be at ease when the abyss yawns beneath him? (And it *does*—the abyss is *there*, most clearly symbolized in the universal destiny of *death*; to pretend that we walk on solid ground is to miss the whole point.) How can a person accept himself and his situation when his own worth, his destiny, and his being are out of control, as far as he is concerned?

Acceptance in faith

We touch a dimension of the struggle of mental illness that is significantly religious.

Deep within every person—in fact at the core of every person—is a yearning for meaning, for wholeness, for enduring value. That yearning leads a person on a lifelong quest, as he seeks his meaning consciously or unconsciously in heaven knows how many different ways, some more and some less appropriate and effective. But no human way gives a meaning that is beyond a doubt, a wholeness that is truly complete, or a value that really endures. The dark side threatens, and the abyss yawns. Left to himself, a person can only see that he cannot ever fulfill his ultimate yearning, and that his quest is ultimately hopeless. Every merely human effort to find meaning is frustrated ultimately by the universal law that all living creatures suffer and die, and all monuments erode and decay. Whatever his laudable efforts toward acceptance, if a person faces the dark side and the abyss alone, there is no foundation for hope, the yearning for meaning at his core remains a useless passion, and to encounter the abyss means to despair.

And yet there is a realm where death and its power is not absolute and ultimate. There is One who is not subject to death and decay, but who gives life. There is One who is meaning, who is wholeness, and who is the enduring ground for all value. There is One who is in himself the goal of a person's quest for meaning, God.

God gives himself to mankind without our deserving, redeems us not because we're upright and respectable but precisely because we are sinners and painfully conscious of the dark side. In Christ God presents to us the gift of resurrection from the dead, not because we're comfortably immortal but because the abyss and the ultimate darkness of death yawns before each of us, and Christ shows that to go *through* that darkness in faith is to enter into glory.

And so perhaps the ability to accept oneself—one's dark side—and to be at ease in the face of the abyss is more than meets the eye. Perhaps unspoken beneath that acceptance is the dimly sensed recognition that the dark side doesn't matter all that much because its power is ultimately *overcome*. We can live with the ambiguity of ourselves because we needn't rely on our own perfection for our value and meaning. And we can face the threats to our very being because they have no more power than the realm of death, and we sense a hope that transcends, reaches beyond death. If it is possible then to hold one's hopes and ideals together with one's undesirable tendencies and so to form an integration that is truly all-embracing, truly healthy, then the power that binds this integration is more than acceptance, it is faith—however explicit or implicit it may be. And if it is possible to stand firm even though the abyss yawns, then the ground on which we stand is no mere surface but the transcendent power of God himself, the ground and source of all being and life.

No miracles

While the religious dimension may be fundamental to the struggle toward wholeness that is faced most acutely by the mentally ill, religious faith is not likely to produce immediate "cures" of mental disorders, or miraculously to erase or prevent any of the stresses or anxieties that lead to mental disorders. Faith does not remove the pain of physical sickness, either—it is no passport from suffering and ambiguity.

And so for instance a person may suffer from a mild neurotic condition—most people have quirks and foibles and aspects of their behavior that puzzle or dismay them. But faith can enable a person to live with himself as he is. One man learned through a mental illness that he simply cannot stand highly stressful situations. And so, for instance, he should never try to take on a job as an air traffic controller or a race car driver. It might have been disturbing to him to accept the fact that his mental stability had limits. But to accept limits is the human condition. And it is possible to put up with a limited situation and a limited self because, thank God, everything does not depend on our having everything under control.

Another person is bothered by the tendency to be a perfectionist—a slightly neurotic tendency. Self-acceptance in faith may not erase the habit of being just a bit too meticulous, or of being a bit tentative in his decisions rather than quick and firm. But it can undo the debilitating sense of inadequacy that lies at the root of this tendency and turns it into a real problem in relationship with other people. Faith does not remove feelings of inadequacy. But it may enable a person to feel quite comfortable being inadequate! Inadequate? Of course I'm inadequate, isn't everybody? A healthy sense of humor—an accepting sense of one's limitations—can turn such a tendency from a worry to a simple character trait that has some good aspects. Granted that this person should not try to work as a short-order cook or a radio disc-jockey, his meticulous patience can serve him well in many ways.

In a way, then, the quirks and foibles—minor neuroses—that mark our limits can be accepted in a spirit something like that with which the person with a handicap accepts his physical condition. This is the way I am, and my calling is to make the best of what I am. I have no obligation to live up to an abstract ideal of "mental health"—mental health for me is to embrace my whole being, dark side included, into one affirmation that may be as unimpressive as a chuckle, but has echoes reaching toward transcendence itself.

Chapter 12

Conclusion:
Christian Sickness As Prophecy

We began our Christian reflections on sickness with an attempt to locate the place that sickness has in a person's life and the place it is given in our society. For the sick person or one close to him, we have seen that sickness can mean a painful disruption of the kind of life most people take for granted, and yet a challenge to deep spiritual renewal. In our society, sickness is given place reluctantly if at all—it is something people would rather not have to notice. But it can be a significant reminder of reality nonetheless. And so the place of sickness is a paradoxical one, a mixed blessing to say the least.

The place of sickness that we have discovered bears a remarkable resemblance to the place in which several Old Testament prophets found themselves. In fact, the figure of the prophet provides a good model for understanding how the various aspects and challenges of sickness that we have pondered fit together, for understanding the significance of sickness.

Portrait Of A Prophet

The popular idea of the prophet pictures a kind of fortune-teller, a person who has the ability to predict future events with accuracy. And since sickness seldom provides a person with such extraordinary powers, it may seem strange to speak of sickness as prophecy. But a thoughtful reading of the prophets of the Old Testament reveals that they wasted few words talking about future events. The Old Testament prophet, rather than being a person who has a mysterious vision of future events, is a person who has a keen insight into present reality. The prophets had the ability to see through the pretensions of kings and the deluded dreams of their society, and to call attention to the real challenges that faced their people. And so they were disturbers of the complacent, prods for conscience. (Needless to say, they were not the most socially acceptable people of their day.) But it was God's call which their warnings embodied, and it was God's unsettling word they felt compelled to speak. To a people wandering from God's way into delusions and dreams, the prophets were sobering reminders of reality.

Jeremiah is about as close as we can come to a "typical prophet." He lived in the seventh century before Christ, and he brought his unsettling message to the people of Jerusalem in the years just before the conquering armies of Babylon destroyed that city and dragged her people off into exile.

Jeremiah had to compete with advertisers (false prophets) who encouraged his society in the pursuit of an earthly paradise, saying "I promise you unbroken peace in this place." (Jeremiah 14:13). In the name of God he challenged that dream and denounced the lazy complacency it produced: "Delusive visions, hollow predictions, daydreams of their own, that is what they prophesy to you." (Jer. 14:14). Jeremiah was realistic enough to know that the days ahead would be challenging, and that no earthly city could promise unbroken peace and happiness. But such a reminder of reality was not quite welcome in the polite society of the time. Jeremiah found himself an outcast.

A remarkable thing about this prophet was that he challenged the people of his day less by his words than by his very way of life. He spurned wealth and comfort, and refused to settle down as if the city could provide a secure home. He was therefore "different," and so became the victim of that curious snobbery of the complacent which accuses the person who challenges them of being "snobbish or elitist," and so rejects him. So in spite of himself Jeremiah suffered a good deal from the misunderstanding of his society. He suffered from continual sickness as well. He could take his whole life into a single lament: "Why is my suffering continual, my wound incurable, refusing to be healed?" (Jer. 15:18). He found no satisfaction (as a smug, self-righteous person might) in his rejection and his suffering. "Woe is me, my mother," he cried, "for you have borne me to be a man of strife and of dissension for all the land." (Jer. 15:10). By his very suffering and rejection he became a sharp reminder that the call to be God's people was not a call to wealth and comfort, not even to spiritual comfort.

Through his suffering Jeremiah himself came to a deeper and purer awareness of God and understood in a more and more vital way the hidden power of God at work in his life, and the mysterious promise of God toward which he called his people. And so Jeremiah accepted his suffering as his mission—as the work that was his part in the design of God for his people. As a result, Jeremiah contributed two profoundly valuable things to his people. One was the significance of his suffering itself. The other was the unique insight into God's plan and God's promise that the hard school of suffering gave him.

When events had proved Jeremiah true, his sufferings were understood and appreciated for what they were: a man giving himself to his people as a reminder of reality. It was probably none other than Jeremiah that a later prophet had in mind when he wrote the songs about God's suffering servant:

> Without beauty, without majesty we saw him,
> no looks to attract our eyes;
> a thing despised and rejected by men,
> a man of sorrows and familiar with suffering.
> And yet ours were the sufferings he bore,
> ours the sorrows he carried. . . .
> (Isaiah 53:2–4).

By his suffering for the people Jeremiah became a prophetic image of one to come—one whose suffering would be more than simply a reminder of reality. For God's suffering servant was ultimately to be Jesus Christ. And the fruit of his suffering was to be a new reality, a reality of grace.

Jeremiah's suffering and his faith in God resulted in an insight into that new reality, an insight that filled Jeremiah with profound hope—not for an earthly paradise, but for a God-given renewal of mankind:

> See, the days are coming—it is the Lord who speaks—when I will make a new covenant with the House of Israel. . . . Deep within them I will plant my Law, writing it on their hearts. Then I will be their God and they shall be my people. There will be no further need for neighbor to try to teach neighbor, of brother to say to brother, "Learn to know the Lord!" No, they will all know me, the least no less than the greatest—it is the Lord who speaks—since I will forgive their iniquity and never call their sin to mind.
>
> (Jer. 31:31–34).

Jeremiah then gives us a picture of what it means to be a prophet, specifically a prophet through suffering. By his very suffering he challenged the complacency of his people—a people caught up in the pursuit of an earthly paradise. Through his suffering he came himself to a deeper and purer relationship with God. And so he was able to provide not only a warning against the illusions of his day, but also a hope for a new order of things, God-given, and free from empty dreams.

The sick person can share to some extent the role of Jeremiah. He is a reminder of reality in a world tempted to live in a dream. He is challenged to profound faith and to spiritual growth. And through his suffering and his faith he can point the way toward a genuinely healthy society.

Reminders of Reality

The conventional idea that sickness is an evil to be avoided or hidden, and the conventional get-well card that arises from that idea, have provided for us a window into our society and our culture. We found there a set of assumptions about what life should be—a whole way of living that we called the pursuit of an earthly paradise.

Further reflection led us to see the shortcomings of that aspect of our culture. In fact, we found a frightening parallel between that and the attempt of men, as described in the Old Testament, to build a greatness for themselves without a thought of God. Trying to achieve meaning, wholeness, value—the "good life"—completely on one's own was considered by the faithful Israelite to be radically sinful, for sin is the condition of the man who relies on himself alone rather than on God.

The complacency which the prophets assailed was precisely that radical sinfulness: the state of sin was reflected then, as now, in the effort of people to create the illusion of a paradise on earth by forgetting or ignoring the universal law that all living creatures suffer and die, and all monuments erode and decay—forgetting or ignoring both the rule of death and the call of God.

We have seen in several instances symptoms that suggest our society is indeed rather unhealthy in this regard. Sick people often find themselves virtually abandoned. The aging discover there is no place for them. The handicapped find they are set apart, distressingly "different." These symptoms suggest that the malaise is rather widespread of seeing sickness as meaningless and so of trying to escape it or hide it.

The same malaise produces a distortion of perception where anything having to do with the preservation of the dream is concerned. It can lead to unreasonable expectations and demands made of (or by) medical professionals. It can result in an astounding blindness to injustices in, for instance, nursing homes for the aged or mental hospitals, a blindness coupled ironically with an indignant sensitivity to things which disturb the smooth surface of suburbia. In its advanced state it cripples common sense and produces contradictions on a small scale like the "law 'n' order" advocate who is not fazed by illegal discrimination or "white-collar crime" in government, or anomalies on a global scale like the paranoia

of armament stockpiling, vast efforts to build fail-safe for-
tresses against the universal law that all living creatures and
human societies suffer, decay, and die.

When one is near to waking, the dream of the pursuit of
paradise reveals that it is truly a nightmare. And when he
wakes, startled he feels about him, looks hard into the
darkness to find some reassuring reminders of reality.

Sickness can have the prophet's role of jarring the dreamer
awake. Sickness is a collision with human limitation, a harsh
and uncompromising reminder of the reality of man's finiteness and of the emptiness of the pursuit of an earthly
paradise. Sickness forces the sick person to come to terms
with the reality of the human condition, and through him
confronts our society with a sign of contradiction, a challenge
to truth.

It is quite easy to avoid that truth. We tend to skate merrily
along like water bugs on the thin, deceptive surface of living,
and never think to let ourselves be immersed in its depth.
Until something disturbs that surface, at least—like sickness.
Then the depths make their claim, and either a person learns
to live more deeply or he drowns.

Sickness suggests that living means more than the smooth
surface. Living includes suffering pain, confronting the ugly
and dealing with it honestly, and going through the bumps,
frustrations and struggles that are part of the process of
growth, change, and deepening. And this process goes on
throughout life—so there is never a valid basis for a complacent sense of "having arrived." Sickness echoes the call of the
prophet, a reminder of reality in a world tempted to live in a
dream.

Faith And Growth

Jeremiah found it rather difficult being a living reminder of
reality. But a significant aspect of his call to be God's prophet
was learning to accept his role and his suffering in a spirit of
faith and hope.

The person whose smooth life is shattered by sickness is called to grow in faith as the prophet was. Rebellion, anger and dismay are natural enough as stages along the way of growth—Jeremiah rebelled, another prophet, Jonah, ran, and Job, the just man who suffered beyond his comprehension, demanded an explanation. None escaped the call of God, and to none was given any explanation beyond the simple fact of God's presence and his faithful love. Such suffering called the prophets and calls the sick to a faith that reaches beyond the evident, too-human measure of goods and evils. They are called to rely on God even though they are for all practical purposes left in the dark. But that very faith, which reaches deeper than the surface, leads a person to a more profound relationship with God, and enables a person to discern in suffering an aspect of the mysterious dealing of God with his people. He begins to recognize there the quiet and anonymous work of sickness teaching, testing, and challenging, making real before his dimly perceiving eyes the faint outlines of Christ's own death and resurrection. So the suffering of Jeremiah became a prophetic image of Christ's work of salvation, and the suffering of the sick can become a real participation in that work—significant suffering that bears the promise of fruitfulness beyond any measure.

Sickness can lead the sufferer through the pattern of letting go of dreams, of emptying oneself and placing oneself in God's hands, that echoes Christ's own death and resurrection. We have seen that the critical challenge of nearly every form of sickness is acceptance. Acceptance is more than resignation, which can be a sullen surrender to inevitable defeat. It is more than abandonment, which no longer hopes for anything. Acceptance hopes—not necessarily for a cure to sickness, but rather for meaning and value in sickness. By acceptance sickness is embraced as *what I am doing now*, and the sick person finds assurance through Christ's suffering that what he is doing is a worthwhile accomplishment.

The challenge of sickness to let go of the too-human measure of the surface of life is most dramatically confronted as a person approaches death. Here to let go means to go into utter darkness with only a hope in God's promise that has no tangible guarantee. And yet such faith can illuminate the darkness for one who is dying, and the prophetic power of such faith is immeasurable.

The capacity to let go, to allow oneself to *be* without fear but in faith, means a capacity to dismantle the defenses most people construct to protect and conceal the truth of their human limitations from themselves and from others. Acceptance bears fruit then in availability, the capacity to open oneself to another person, and to leave one's own world behind enough to understand another person genuinely. Availability is itself prophetic, for it testifies to the faith at its root. Perhaps that is one reason that love was to be the distinguishing mark of one who believed in Jesus: "By this love you have for one another, everyone will know you are my disciples." (John 13:35).

A subtle and difficult aspect of accepting human limitations in faith is the challenge posed by a difficult ethical decision. Often people who seek to live by faith are distressed when they face a decision without a clearly defined idea of the right and wrong of it. It takes a more profound faith to act where there are no clear do's and don'ts, but only the call to responsible decision. One's goodness is no longer quite so much under his own control, and he must rely on God without any basis for justifying himself or making a claim on God. Prevented from playing the role of the Pharisee, he finds he is the Publican. The anguish of such a decision is real. But it is a call to a faith profound enough to trust completely in the free—i.e. unearned—gift of grace. The Publican went home visited by God, as the story goes on to say.

Sickness and the suffering connected with it can therefore lead a person to a profound faith in God, one gradually purified of efforts to save himself by his own powers, i.e. purified of sin. And so sickness can bring a person to an awareness of the presence of God to him, and to an understanding of the power of God at work in his life.

Pointing The Way

Christian sickness can raise a prophetic question to a society permeated by the dreamy pursuit of paradise. And the sick person can come to accept his sickness and so develop a profound faith. But from this prophetic questioning and this prophetic faith there can come, indirectly, slowly, a whole new way of looking at the world. Sickness awakens a person from the pursuit of an earthly paradise where everything is apparently under control and there are no unpleasant surprises. But in its place a wholly different vision can arise, one of authentic health, and of realistic Christian hope.

As the sick person struggles to understand and accept his condition, he will have to turn from the dreamy pursuit of paradise that believes sickness is in itself worthless and meaningless, and he will find a place for sickness that allows it to contribute its significance to the meaning of his life. In that turning he will be reaching toward an authentic health, which makes of all the bits and pieces of life a unified sense, a harmonious whole, and gives significance to every aspect of life, even sickness.

One noteworthy shift in perspective may well have to do with how a person understands himself in relation to the human community in which he lives. The dream of earthly paradise promises to each individual a private Eden—perhaps a self-contained family unit in a private home on a landscaped and measured plot in the suburbs. And part of the promise is bodily and mental integrity: there can't be anything wrong with me in my Eden. But sickness impresses on a person the fragility of the individual person's hopes and dreams, and as well how interdependent human beings really are. No one can stand alone. And so gradually a sick person can discover meaning, wholeness, and a sense of enduring value not in himself alone but in his union and solidarity with the human community under God. It doesn't *really* matter then if he is "different," for the human community finds value and richness precisely in diversity, and in the varied roles, contributions, and burdens that make it up. He knows that he has a contribution to make, that his sickness has real value for it is a share of the human burden to bear for the sake of his fellowmen. The "rugged individualist" living in an earthly paradise is shaken from his slumber by sickness. And in his place rises a new image of mankind: a people *sharing* life, its blessings and its burdens; a people who are *on the way*, and on the way *together*.

But toward what are we on our way? There is an expectation, a hope that gives direction and meaning to our struggle and our progress.

That hope is given shape by the Christian faith. With Jesus all humanity was given a way to freedom from the realm where a person is left to himself in empty delusions, a way to the realm of God, the reality of grace, where a person can discover the free gift of God's love and can find himself embraced within the people of God, a pilgrim people. The hope of Christian believers is for the universal completion of the realm of God—the coming of the perfect kingdom ruled by Christ, the final day of fulfillment when the design of God is complete, for "all things to be reconciled through him and for him, everything in heaven and everything on earth." (Colossians 1:20).

Christian hope denies nothing of the sorrow and frustration of human existence. Suffering is real. Sickness is no pleasure. Death holds a real reason for terror. But in the face of these harsh realities Christian hope affirms that a greater power is at work to restore and renew, to purify and make clear, to complete and perfect. And it is not a pie-in-the-sky heaven that the Christian hopes for, a misty place to which each individual ascends upon his death to receive his own personal harp and halo. Rather he hopes for the renewal and fulfillment of the earth itself and its people, the resurrection of these very bodies that are the place where we now find ourselves, and the completion and perfection of human community. The Christian hopes for himself to contribute to and share in the coming of that kingdom.

> Then I saw a new heaven and a new earth. . . . I saw the holy city, the new Jerusalem, coming down from God out of heaven, as beautiful as a bride all dressed for her husband. Then I heard a loud voice call from the throne, "You see this city? Here God lives among men. He will make his home among them; they shall be his people, and he will be their God; his name is God-with-them. He will wipe away all tears from their eyes; there will be no more death, and no more mourning or sadness. The world of the past has gone." Then the One sitting on the throne spoke: "Now I am making the whole of creation new."
>
> (Revelations 21:1–8).

This is the shape of the Christian hope that points the way along which mankind can walk together. Filled with such hope, the Christian has reason to be eager for the coming of that promise, and to be enthusiastic to contribute to its coming by his work and his suffering in the present time.

For in the light of this hope, the apparent frustrations and the acute or long drawn-out suffering of sickness takes on an extremely important meaning. This hope has substance because of the death and resurrection of Christ, which has established the kingdom and overcome the realm of death. Our suffering now shares in Christ's suffering, indeed brings his suffering to fruitfulness. St. Paul gave us this insight:

> It makes me happy to suffer for you, as I am suffering now, and in my own body to make up all that has still to be undergone by Christ for the sake of his body, the Church.
>
> (Colossians 1:24).

So the hidden work of sickness is a share in bringing the people of God closer to their fulfillment. Sickness is no solitary challenge, but it can be for *others*, though that is something hidden in the present time. The sick person does not have the ego-flattering satisfaction of actually seeing the benefit of his suffering, as if it were something he accomplished wholly on his own. It is the power of God at work in his suffering that gives meaning to what would otherwise appear useless. He can only present himself to God, doing what is his to do and hoping in God for the value of it.

Sickness then has a place within the Christian vision of the world, indeed a significant place in relation to the coming of the kingdom of God. All suffering and sickness can be a share in the whole world's longing and so it can be fruitful labor toward the day of fulfillment—the labor of giving life:

> I think that what we suffer in this life can never be compared to the glory, as yet unrevealed, which is waiting for us. The whole creation is eagerly waiting for God to reveal his sons. . . . Creation still retains the hope of being freed, like us, from its slavery to decadence, to enjoy the same freedom and glory as the children of God. From the beginning until now the entire creation, as we know, has been groaning in one great act of giving birth; and not only creation, but all of us who possess the first-fruits of the spirit, we too groan inwardly as we wait for our bodies to be set free.
>
> (Romans 8:18–23).